THE NEW AMERICANS:

DEFINING OURSELVES THROUGH SPORTS AND FITNESS PARTICIPATION

* * * *

HARVEY LAUER

American Sports Data, Inc.

www.americansportsdata.com

Copyright © 2006 by Harvey Lauer. All rights reserved. No part of this book may be used or produced by any means, graphic, electronic, or mechanical, including photocopying, recording, taping or by any information storage retrieval system without the written permission of the publisher.

Published by American Sports Data, Inc.
www.americansportsdata.com
ISBN 0-9779079-0-2
Designed by Kenneth E. Kaufman
Printed in the United States of America

THE NEW AMERICANS:
DEFINING OURSELVES THROUGH SPORTS AND FITNESS PARTICIPATION

* * *

TABLE OF CONTENTS

Dedication v
Acknowledgements vi
Foreward ix
Introduction 1

Part One: Interviews

1. The Lauer Report: Insight from Statistics 27
2. A CBI Interview with Harvey Lauer 31
3. A Health & Fitness Business Interview with Harvey Lauer 41

Part Two: Physical Fitness

4. Grandparents Fitter than Grandchildren? 51
5. The New Fitness Mantras: Flexibility and Strength 59
6. The Gap between Attitudes and Behavior:
   Four Levels of Fitness Consciousness 67
7. Health Club Strategy for the New Millennium:
   The Pursuit of Consciousness III 75
8. Psychological Stress: Invisible Public Health Enemy Number One 87
9. Kinder, Gentler Exercise: The Democratization of Physical Fitness 95
10. The Future of Fitness 103
11. Fitness *and* Fatness Boom: The New American Paradox 107
12. Nationwide Health Concerns may be Pumping U.S. Behavior 121
13. A New Front in the War on Obesity 129
14. Contrarian Philosophies: Fat is Okay -- Especially If You're Fit 133
15. The Weight Loss Wars: Advantage…Health Clubs 139
16. Older Americans Drive Physical Fitness 147
17. Physical Fitness -- A Thumbnail History 155
18. Wave of the Future: The Subsidization of Physical Fitness 163

Part Three: Sports Participation

19. "Extreme Sports" Bonanza 179
20. Current Issues in Youth Sports 189
21. Sports Participation: The Metaphor of Youth Development 199
22. New Millennial Pursuits Outpace Traditional Sports 211
23. The Stereotype of "Generation Y" 221
24. The Great Outdoors Revolution: Lifestyle or State of Mind? 227
25. Sports Injuries: The Neglected Stepchild of Research 235
26. Sports Injuries in the U.S. 245
27. Hunting, Shooting and Social Analysis 251

Part Four: Research Issues

28. The Primacy of Sports Participation Research 261
29. Interpreting Sports Participation Research 267
30. Sports Participation Research: Not Yet a Science 275
31. Point-of-Sale (POS) Research in the Sporting Goods Industry 293
32. A Consumer Mail Panel Research Methodology for
    Surveying Ethnic Populations 297
33. You Say Evolution, I Say Devolution 303

Appendix: The Superstudy® Of Sports Participation (1987 - 2004) 317

Index 329

Personal Dedications

To Sandra, my wife of 33 years, who breathes life and truth into all the old clichés. She put me through college, through graduate school, bore and raised my children, runs my business, and typed every word I ever wrote -- including this book. And now, she still has the patience to look after me in very young Old Age...

To my first-born son Russell, greatest superachiever of all time. Though he does not share my love of numbers, his 2:45 marathon and 4.0 GPA very much gratify my love of numerical achievement. He can succeed at anything he chooses, and is destined for big things.

To my son Dorian, who has inherited my love of the language, his mother's character, her work ethic and a passion that has already carried him to the heights of his profession. If given the opportunity, he will revolutionize modern sportscasting.

To my clone-baby, Erin, who is also capable of anything she undertakes. Wherever you are, we love you....

PROFESSIONAL ACKNOWLEDGEMENTS

I have always believed that for the most part, our abilities descend directly from DNA, and our achievements from nurture. Sociobiologists will someday provide better answers about human nature; but we can never really acknowledge our external influences, because nurture, in a word, is unknowable. Outside of biology, we will never know who or what made us, and in what proportions.

With this grand disclaimer, I claim Henry James, Oscar Wilde, Tom Wolfe and other great thinkers, writers and social analysts who have, quite ineffably, contributed to the piece of work that is me. These are my unknowable Walter Mitty influences.

In real life, I acknowledge Daniel Yankelovich, founder and guiding spirit of the Public Agenda Foundation, giant of 20th century social research, and (though he never knew) by far my greatest professional influence. My fondest memories of the early Public Agenda Foundation were our quotidian drills of the late 1970's…

> …"A chart should say just one thing."
> …"If you haven't done five drafts, it's not worth a shit!"
> …"Jean, that doesn't look like two pounds…bring me my scale!"

It was the best Boot Camp a fledgling researcher ever had, and I hope kids there today are getting the same training.

I am grateful also to Martin Duberman, the only other big name I ever knew up close. Already a celebrated author, playwright and Distinguished Professor of History at City College in the early 1970's, later a leading intellectual and activist of the Gay Rights Movement, Duberman was also a pioneer of "radical" teaching methods. It was probably in one of his early "touchy-feely" seminars -- the effects of which lingered a full week -- until the next class -- that I first became acquainted with the word "humanistic".

I thank Vickie Karp for her help over the years. She is a personal friend, prize-winning poet, and the only one ever allowed to see my rough scribbling. Like me, she aspires only to posthumous recognition…

To Kerry E. Smith, Old Amigo, running partner, whose opinion is one of the few I ever cared about. He is my gold standard for hyperlogical thinking.

Sebastian DiCasoli, loyal friend, best gatekeeper SGMA ever had, and who more than anyone, helped perpetuate my research. Special thanks to the Sporting Goods Manufacturers Association, long-time sponsor of the Superstudy®, without whose support this body of knowledge would probably not exist.

To Walter Fackner of Crosstabs, Inc., last of a vanishing breed, who for more than 20 years tolerated my perfectionistic excesses -- because he knows what it takes to be the best. I hope we produce a few more like him, but I doubt it…

To John McCarthy, Executive Director of the International Health, Racquet & Sportsclub Association (IHRSA) for more than a quarter century -- the best friend anyone could ever hope for, and in my opinion, defining figure of the American health club industry in the 20th century.

* * *

FOREWARD

For every student of American sports and fitness participation, whether they study it from an academic perspective or whether they are involved in sports and fitness marketing, this collection of articles and essays by Harvey Lauer is a must read.

No one has a more comprehensive grasp, nor does anyone have a more incisive understanding of the trends and movements underlying American sports and fitness participation than Harvey Lauer. The text is a comprehensive, quantum advance for sports sociology: It brings the reader to the unique confluence of sports participation and social analysis.

A student of the great societal analyst Daniel Yankelovich, Lauer brings to this volume all the multi-disciplinary tools of social and behavioral analysis necessary to decipher where and why fitness and sports participation is where it is today, and where it is likely to be in the future. This book traverses every conceivable aspect of sports and fitness -- history, contemporary social analysis, sports injuries, Generation Y, health clubs, obesity, research methodology -- everything. His command of the subject matter is surpassing.

Since 1987, when IHRSA (the International Health, Racquet, and Sportsclub Association) first engaged Harvey Lauer to help us understand how, when, and where the market for fitness services was likely to grow, he has been an invaluable and irreplaceable asset to the entire worldwide fitness industry.

Even more importantly, he has invariably pointed us in the right direction in terms of future growth opportunities in the various age, economic, and gender segments of the marketplace.

This seminal book is destined to become the *Merck's Manual* for everyone who needs to understand what needs to be done to increase sports and fitness participation in America.

Given the multiple and serious health conditions that we now know to be associated with sedentary living, this text could not have been published at a more opportune time.

John McCarthy
Executive Director, IHRSA
Boston, Massachusetts
March 2006

INTRODUCTION

When I started a marketing research business a quarter century ago, I intuited that sports participation might be a crude sociological mirror of the larger society. I soon came to believe that after religion, "sport" is not only the most powerful force in American culture -- but also a precision index of changing values and behavioral norms.

Sports participation statistics are of interest to a great number of individuals and organizations who regularly seek information on populations of sports participants: how many people play, how often, demographic profiles, geography, cross-participation, attitudes, motivations and other characteristics. These numbers find a wide variety of practical and theoretical applications: sporting goods market research, business plans, sports event marketing, health club research, fitness trend forecasting, public health assessment, sports injury epidemiology, tourism, advertising and rarely -- academic inquiries into the nature of cultural change.

This volume is <u>not</u> about professional teams, celebrity athletes, or any facets of spectatorship that are commonly associated with "sports". It focuses on a far more important phenomenon: everyday sports and fitness <u>participation</u> by ordinary people. It is a collection of thirty-three pieces written over a five-year period (2000 - 2005). There are three published interviews, twelve press releases, twelve essays, four snippets extracted from research reports, and two published articles. All are somehow related to primary research conducted by American Sports Data, Inc. -- a business I formed in 1983 for the purpose of conducting sports marketing research.

In the late 1990's, two things happened that would result in the ultimate publication of this book. First, I would become bored with numbers...a vacuum eventually filled by writing. Second, I would be swept up by the Internet revolution.

The Internet revolution demanded a website, and the new website required appealing copy. Inevitably, this new phase rekindled a latent interest in social research that took root many years earlier as a student of Daniel Yankelovich at the New School for Social Research, original home to the fledgling Public Agenda Foundation -- a public policy research organization founded by Yankelovich and Cyrus Vance in 1975. As a part-time graduate student, I became charter employee, whereupon followed my baptism in social analysis -- a lifelong fascination.

In 2005, I decided there would be a book, and it would be easy, because the collection was mostly written; all that remained was some polishing and a brief introduction. The task was simple. I needed only enumerate or summarize -- not analyze -- the wide array of topics I had written about over the last five or six years. The diverse subject matter would run the entire gamut of sports participation, including varied and often unrelated issues such as sports participation trends, injuries, obesity, psychological stress, the history of fitness, Generation Y, shooting sports, youth devel-

Introduction

opment, methodology and so on. I needed only a straightforward introduction to impose some order on a wide-ranging mosaic of writings.

But in the end -- as I knew it would -- the pull of social analysis became irresistible. So rather than a simple, straightforward summary of the book's content, this introductory piece began to veer toward sports sociology. I needed to connect the dots.

A DEFINITION OF HUMANISTIC EVOLUTION

Many social themes emerge from 25 years of sports participation research. Some leap right off the page, while others are more subtle and ambiguous -- subject to interpretation, or demanding to be teased out by careful social analysis. But one idea towers majestically above all others, surfacing repeatedly as a major correlate of sports participation behavior. In the present context, this psychosocial theme is utterly secular, having absolutely nothing to do with the philosophy of humanism or any raging religious controversy of the same name. I have selected a provocative phrase that will draw much unwanted mail, and with America straining at the leash, one that is outrageously counterintuitive. But there is no better description of this unmistakable grand theme: it is *humanistic evolution*.

The first decade of the New Millennium -- both in societal values and official policy -- is the counterculture on steroids. From the mundane to the momentous -- from taking our dog to work, to anti-gun legislation, to gay marriage, to interracial dating, to the first real prospect of a female president -- the imprint of humanistic evolution is undeniable.

There is a tremendous complexity and ambivalence in what Daniel Yankelovich calls the "New Social Morality". A great dilemma according to Yankelovich, is that "the rise in social tolerance has gone hand in hand with a weakening social morality". Perhaps tolerance and morality are two sides of the same coin....maybe we can't have one without the other. We cherish our new tolerance, but paradoxically, long for a return to certain traditional values.

For me, humanistic social evolution betokens a growing awareness -- an ongoing process of developing human potential, of becoming more enlightened about ourselves, our planet, the environment, our bodies, our relationships, and less beholden to authority and formality in all its guises. But the current zeitgeist of anger, strife, polarization and yearning for a bygone era create an ambiguity that seems almost irreconcilable; yet, the march of social progress shines through 25 years of sports and fitness research, and appears inexorable.

What drives humanistic evolution? Aside from the natural, mystical imperative that governs all evolution, a more obvious stimulant is economics -- the clichéd rising tide. The lifting of all boats in a progressively richer economy (also the most elegant explanation for a plunging crime rate) has facilitated a far more tolerant, permissive and humanistic society than was possible forty years ago.

Introduction

Psychological constructs such as ego, acquisitiveness and aggression may be immutable human constants, not subject to evolution -- humanistic or otherwise. But this is not at issue, and even if it were, such profound genetic alterations could not occur in the evolutionary eye-blink of a generation or two. In the present context, humanistic evolution is about changes in social values and collective thinking, and how the rules of society -- written and unwritten -- are being transformed.

A state-of-the-art template -- made of tolerance, personal values, individual freedom and a social benevolence unprecedented in American History -- has been under construction for about 50 years. In some sense, it is the cultural revolution of the 1960's fast-forwarded to 2006 -- the ideals of permissiveness, diversity, pluralism, personal freedom, individualism, self-fulfillment, sensitivity and altruism -- minus all the original mistakes, excesses, and wrong-headedness. The legacy of the counterculture is everywhere, but it co-exists with the crudeness, incivility and aggression that typify our daily experience.

A COUNTERINTUITIVE NOTION

The current political environment in the U.S. makes few concessions to any form of humanism. From a global perspective, the proposition becomes even more untenable, for history will not be kind to the 20th century. It was after all, scene of the bloodiest genocidal rampages ever, an era of unbridled aggression, militarism, unremitting greed and toward the end -- midwife to world terrorism.

Critics need not wait for the judgments of history, for they see ample refutation in the present. Children are being raised on video games that openly promote violence; ethical standards are being demolished by corporate role models; violence and sex fill our media and entertainment cultures; and uncivil social behavior -- epitomized by road rage, offensive cell-phone usage, brazen graffiti defacement, rambunctious and sometimes violent fan behavior at professional sports events -- makes everyday living nearly intolerable. These are the major symptoms of a weakened social morality, the natural culmination of a decades-long erosion of authority, or more fancifully -- the pent-up tensions of a conflicted society, ignited by the events of 9/11.

Moving closer to home, but still far from the subject matter -- to the tarnished venue of professional sports teams and celebrity athletes -- humanistic evolution becomes an even more dubious abstraction. Rather than "giving back" -- the traditional credo of the celebrity athlete -- today's subculture of anti-heroes has given us a legacy of violence, sexual misconduct, dishonesty and steroids…with extravagant, undeserved paychecks the final insult. *But celebrity athletes have little to do with participant sports…*

This brutal indictment is largely anecdotal, but it rings true. On the other hand, there is also (better-documented) survey evidence that Americans are decidedly sympathetic toward religion, charity, social welfare and children. This is not to mention a half century of heightened social tolerance, growing rights movements and wildly proliferating entitlement legislation.

Paradoxically, the infamous 20th century was also the most glorious; it lavished upon us colossal advances in health, wealth, longevity, and quality-of-life, not to mention the greatest unsolved sociological riddle in American history -- a plummeting crime rate. For America and most of the planet, the 20th century was exponential progress; but whether or not the world became a better place will be debated for many decades.

EVIDENCE FROM SPORTS PARTICIPATION

It is difficult to see at the moment, especially against the glare of current events; but through the lens of sports and fitness participation, the grand theme of humanistic evolution is clear and unmistakable. This new social scaffolding -- which ranges far beyond mere tolerance for diversity -- is supported by at least 10 sports and fitness phenomena:

1. Decline of the "Blood" Sports
2. Changing perceptions of Women's athleticism and sexual attractiveness
3. New attitudes toward Senior Fitness
4. Tolerance of the Obesity Subculture
5. The Fitness Revolution
6. A heightened Outdoors Consciousness
7. The War on Smoking
8. Title IX

9. Sports Safety
10. The Subsidization of Physical Fitness

Of these ten topics, four deal with social tolerance (caring about others), three with personal welfare (caring about ourselves), and one each with animal rights, social welfare, and the environment.

Lest I be guilty of cherry-picking, various other questions, obstacles and competing explanations are explored. They include: Obesity, the Sedentary Lifestyle, the Me-Generation and Extreme Sports. Several other topics contained in this volume -- notably Youth Development, Technology, Sports Injuries, Sports Iconography and the Trend Toward Informality -- may be regarded as "neutral".

Humanistic growth is revealed most poignantly in the "Blood" sports -- the demise of which, over the last several decades, are the most compelling testimony.

Women, and older exercisers are among the once-excluded groups also offering powerful support for this idea. So commonplace and mainstream are these constituencies that in a contemporary discussion of the Fitness culture, their mere mention seems gratuitous.

The Fitness Revolution itself is a ringing testimonial to a never-ending obsession with our bodies, much of it health-related. To this extent, it is also a monument to an evolved human condition, but the evidence is not unanimous, because we have two uncooperative witnesses: the sedentary lifestyle and an obesity epidemic. And, some will say, Fitness has selfish roots: it springs from the Me-Generation. But these semantic muddles of obesity, selfishness and fitness are not refutations.

For example, the Obesity epidemic does not signal a reversal of health and Fitness values; people are not returning to some slothful, dissolute way of life. As a major essay explains, Obesity has many causes, and remarkably, the vast majority of overweight Americans are very health-conscious; a small number are "constitutionally" over-sized, but most are simply bereft of self-discipline. Half of the U.S. population tried to shed poundage in 2004, including 68% of those who were overweight.

Like racial, ethnic, female, older, gay and disabled minorities, the obesity subculture is protected by the shield of political correctness and other expressions of tolerance and social support, such as recent Medicare legislation sanctifying Obesity as a disease. These are not contradictions, but clear manifestations of the paradigm shift.

All revolutions have logical problems, and the "Great Outdoors Revolution" is no exception. Gardening, day visits to state parks, bird watching, organic food consumption and other "eco" pursuits are at an all-time high; yet, as a full-blown essay will demonstrate, vigorous Outdoors sports participation is in decline. The discrepancy between a highly-developed Outdoors Consciousness and lagging

Outdoors sports participation is analogous to the ironic coexistence of a Fitness Revolution and Obesity Epidemic. Both paradoxes have the same root -- a perennial lack of discipline. People love the Outdoors but are participating less in Outdoors sports; we are also very health-conscious, yet have motivational problems with exercise and dieting. In both arenas, a lack of discipline co-exists uneasily with an elevated consciousness.

Less ambiguous testimony is provided by the eradication of smoking -- a grindingly slow but resounding argument for humanistic evolution.

My case for tolerance, altruism and social improvement is not exhaustive; it omits the compulsory use of crash helmets, face masks, protective equipment, and a host of other sports safely rules and regulations which have spared many grievous injuries and saved countless lives. It mentions but does not amplify the historic 1972 Title IX legislation, landmark in the annals of gender equity.

BLOOD SPORTS

Nowhere is the imprint of humanistic evolution more apparent than in the so-called Blood Sports. In 2003, there were 40% fewer Hunters in the U.S. than in 1987 -- and if not for population expansion, the fall would have been steeper. From 1982 - 2001, Rifle and Shotgun manufacture in the U.S. declined by 21% and 23% respectively, while Handgun production plummeted by 64%. And contrary to the illusions of its opponents, NRA membership has eroded from a peak of 4.3 million in 2000, to 3.4 million in 2003. Fishing is still largest of the genre, but even this most benign Blood Sport has declined by 9% since 1987. Changing social values are not the only factors, but they are pre-eminent.

Outside the U.S., a ban on Professional Boxing has existed in Sweden since 1970, while a similar prohibition in China dates to 1949. In most of the world, the truly hideous anachronisms of Cockfighting and Dogfighting face imminent extinction.

In America, more socially acceptable diversions, including Target Shooting (where animals are not killed or wounded), are more respectable. The "Bloodless" Bullfight (still deemed barbaric), Sporting Clays (substituting projectiles for birds and small animals) and Paintball (which replaces bullets with harmless paint pellets) are at least stable -- or gaining in popularity.

DEMOGRAPHICS AND CHANGING VALUES
Forty years ago, over-sized bosoms were the rage... Remember Miss Wall Street? In the fifties and sixties a well-toned, ever-so-slightly-muscular woman was a vaguely freakish anomaly.

It took 40 or 50 years, but the male psyche has undergone a fundamental transformation; for many, the slender, toned woman represents an ideal of sexual attractiveness. And for some time, women have been permitted the joys of sweating -- even the privilege of growing firm muscles! Today, female Strength-Training is one of the fastest rising Fitness activities; from 1987 - 2004 Free Weight training for women had increased by 236%, compared with 86% for men. For many men and women, it is true that exercise has more to do with simply "looking good" than with the "pure" motives of health and fitness. But in their quest for exercise -- in their <u>right</u> to exercise -- women have achieved parity with men. This is a smashing victory for humanistic evolution.

Older people share a similar tale of physical liberation. If in the 1950's, one of our grandmothers looked out the kitchen window and saw a gray-haired man running through the streets in his "underwear"…would she not have called the police?? Just several decades ago, such a sight was at best, faintly deviant; at worst, capable of producing hysteria. Now, it is commonplace.

In striking parallel to the evolution of female fitness, changing social norms and perceptions have dramatically advanced senior participation. Exercise for older people is not merely socially acceptable but fervently encouraged -- a values change that in concert with a new, huge subtrend of medical and therapeutic referral is responsible for the emergence of Kinder/Gentler fitness activities such as Pilates, Yoga, Hand Weights, Treadmills and Recumbent Cycling. Since 1987, overall health club membership has increased by a very robust +138%; but for people over 55, the statistical news is even better: this vital fitness demographic has skyrocketed by 563%! According to other ASD findings, senior citizens are literally buoying the Fitness Movement.

This paradigm shift has nothing to do with the athletic prowess of older men; it is our *acceptance* of older men running through the streets in their underwear!

INTERPRETING FITNESS MOTIVATION

It can be imagined that the Fitness Revolution -- arguably one of the most profound values changes in American history and the quintessential example of caring about our bodies -- is the <u>essence</u> of a new humanistic framework. But this is only a half-truth, because while the Fitness Movement satisfies the definition in one sense -- as a loftier, more idealistic expression of human development -- it can also be seen as anything but humanistic: a selfish derivative of an entirely selfish phenomenon -- the Me-Generation.

The 1970's was the decade in which many of the 1960's counterculture values spilled over into the American mainstream. The new concern about physical fitness was only one manifestation of Self-Fulfillment -- a megatrend that spawned the health food craze, a psychological self-help genre, a cult of self-expression, an ethos of sexual freedom and a host of other movements that focused on the indulgence, pleasure, fulfillment and well-being of the <u>individual</u>.

Caring about "my health" is not quite the same as caring about "my body"....and neither is synonymous with the right to "express myself" or "be me"; but the Fitness Revolution embodies all these ideas, and its genealogy is both humanistic and ego-driven, a duality that does not compromise our general proposition.

THE WAR ON SMOKING

It claims an even earlier pedigree, so the War on Smoking is not a selfish descendant of the Me-Generation; it is arguably the greatest behavioral triumph in the history of American public health. Between 1979 and 2002, adult smoking in the U.S. declined by one-third, a victory attributable not to the narcissistic culture of the 1970's -- but to humanistic evolution.

ASD has drawn an historic parallel between the present Obesity epidemic and the War on Smoking. 40 years after the landmark 1964 Surgeon General's Report, the incidence of adult smoking has been slashed dramatically, and -- the current blip in youth behavior notwithstanding -- may well be on the road to extinction. Some feel that in the war on Obesity, history will be repeated.

Others say it's easier to *quit smoking* than to *restrict eating*. People could simply *stop* smoking -- an indulgence found eventually to be deadly. The U.S. population however, is not yet convinced that overeating can be lethal; nor can people just stop eating -- a powerful human instinct which happens also to provide one of life's greatest pleasures. But to level the playing field, overeaters have an antidote unavailable to smokers -- physical activity.

THE FITNESS PARADOX

A half-century ago, still concerned with "survival" -- or by then "appearance" issues -- unevolved Americans were innocent of psychological fulfillment, preventive healthcare or other "higher concerns". Today, over 80% of the adult population is Health and Fitness-conscious, though only about 1 out of 5 gets enough exercise -- a paradox explaining the awkward coexistence of an Obesity epidemic with a highly-developed awareness of Physical Fitness. In this early phase of our evolution, behavior simply lags enlightened attitudes.

From a near-zero baseline in the 1950's, the Fitness phenomenon grew to 51.5 million frequent participants in 1990 -- a plateau upon which it languished for more than a decade. The chief adversary of fitness is most likely the "Pleasure Principle". In its true incarnation, the latter is something more complex; but in common parlance, the Pleasure Principle refers simply to the seeking of pleasure and the avoidance of pain. Exercise is time-consuming, inconvenient, even painful; and while it offers certain pleasures, attractions, and is said even to cause addictions - - on balance, it is rife with motivational obstacles and avoided by most Americans. Small wonder that Health Clubs and Personal Trainers -- benefiting from a massive failure of self-motivation -- have flourished in the face of "flat" Fitness behavior.

On the other hand, if we extrapolate the logarithmic curve of Fitness to the year 2050, we arrive at the utopian scenario in which people have conquered all motivational obstacles, and every able-bodied American exercises every day. Those who do not are viewed a "pariahs" -- akin to the misfits who did not brush their teeth every day back in 2006!

But right now, Americans admit they can't do it on their own, and are primed to receive even more help from Health Clubs, Personal Trainers, and as we shall see -- the nascent phenomenon of incentivized Physical Fitness.

OBESITY

In this context, Obesity is a confusing theme; it seems to cut both ways into a theory of "humanistic evolution". Except for the CDC, American Sports Data, Inc. is the only research entity to "weigh the nation". In both 2003 and 2004, roughly 4 million Americans tipped the scales at 300 pounds. In 2004, the average adult female weighed in at 165 pounds, as men climbed to a mean bodyweight of nearly 200. A combination of poor eating habits and physical inactivity has produced a grotesque sideshow in which the term "Ugly American" -- formerly a political epithet -- is invested with a new symbolism.

The U.S. Obesity epidemic however, does not necessarily contradict an ethos of health-consciousness. Analogous to the second deadly sin of physical inactivity, overeating merely represents a second massive failure of self-motivation. 4 out of 5 Americans are fitness-conscious; fully half

Introduction

(50%) tried to lose weight in 2004. So the condition of Obesity, in and of itself, is not the indifference of a dissolute populace -- but the flagging resolve of a well-intentioned nation. We <u>care deeply</u> about Physical Fitness; we just can't muster the discipline to restrict eating and exercise sufficiently -- another ironic counterpoint to our enlightened consciousness.

In a recent development, Obesity has been sanctioned by Medicare as a bona fide disease -- entitling patients so diagnosed (under certain conditions) to prescription drugs, doctor's visits and other benefits which were previously deemed frivolous, indulgent or otherwise inapplicable.

The Obesity subculture is one of the last bastions of social injustice which -- because of primal biases buried deep in our national psyche -- has yet to receive the redress finally afforded ethnic, racial, female, older, gay and disabled minorities. The issue is complex, and this subculture itself is not without responsibility; but in terms of <u>accepting</u> Obesity and supporting the rights of this group, the positive imprint of humanistic evolution is clearly visible. <u>Combating</u> Obesity is a different struggle.

A NEW CASUAL WORLD

In part, humanistic development has been defined as growing enlightenment -- about our bodies, our relationships with others and about our environment. Sports and fitness participation are important components of this progress, moving on a parallel evolutionary path with larger societal issues: animal rights movements, capital punishment, penology, environmental concerns, human rights, job safety, health protection, and so on.

Another pillar of humanistic evolution is a new worldview; a less rigid, more relaxed, more casual attitude toward authority, language, entertainment, social formality, and most prominently -- dress and clothing. Most sports apparel and athletic footwear are non-functional, have never witnessed perspiration, and have little to do with Physical Fitness. However, they have much in common with this second tier of humanistic norms -- the relaxation of authority, social hierarchy and decorum.

These have been the major testimonials to humanistic evolution in sports participation, but the theme will surface again. The remainder of this introduction brings us to other interstices of sports and social trends -- some of which are unrelated to our major thesis.

SPORTS ICONOGRAPHY

A need for comfort and the rejection of formality are not the only inspirations of sports fashion; casual clothing styles are driven also by a powerful, well-exploited consumer need for identification. Surfwear, camouflage, safari vests, ski parkas, cargo pants, backpacks, hiking boots, and Hummers are all examples of what I have elsewhere termed "Rugged Chic".

Thematic streetwear, other Outdoors symbols, and the growing popularity of less taxing activities such as bird watching, organic gardening, or sightseeing at national parks, etc. all reflect a primal Outdoors consciousness. But this mindset has nothing to do with <u>actual Outdoors sports participation</u> -- a phenomenon in *severe decline.*

Less strenuous, more cerebral connections with nature and the outdoors appear to be flourishing. They may be hard-wired, or indeed reflect humanistic evolution; but more rigorous expressions of this same root dynamic (Hiking, Camping and Mountain Biking) are withering. American attitudes toward nature bespeak a highly-developed Outdoors sensitivity…but one that is revealed only in lifestyle symbolism, spectatorship or other physically undemanding behavior. Here, evidence for humanistic evolution may be found on more contemplative levels, not in rigorous Outdoor behavior.

The disconnect between attitude and behavior is not without precedent, and certainly not limited to Rugged Outdoors sports. Those old enough to remember the Fitness Boom of the early 1970's recall not only the physical goals of the new movement but also its early iconography. Nylon running suits worn as everyday streetwear came to depict a superior breed which exercised not only for the tangible goal of fitness -- but for the new, higher motives of self-expression and self-fulfillment.

This was also the golden age of the "Velour Runner", found on the sidelines of the New York City marathon in the late 1970's -- the overweight ancestor of today's sedentary emulator. Urban anthropologists have uncovered distinctive recognition markers of these forerunners: dangling cigarettes, mint-condition uniforms; expensive headbands, colorful velour running suits, heretofore unused (and very pricey) $130 New Balance running shoes. The velour is gone, but the subspecies thrives. On rare occasions, their descendants can be sighted running through hallways of Manhattan high-rises, "in training" for the bloated, commercialized extravaganza that is now the New York City Marathon.

Somewhat analogously, about the same time, a bicycle clip on the right pant leg became an ecological status symbol -- no less a political statement than granny glasses, Perrier or the ritualistic consumption of Crunchy Granola.

EXTREME SPORTS AND TRADITIONAL SPORTS: NEW vs. OLD VALUES

Generation "Y" -- whatever the category signifies -- is true to its reputation of disdain; it does not cooperate with our central thesis.

Consider the stereotype of an angry, nose-ringed Skateboarder, replete with tattoos, colored hair, and of course, the most prominent testimonial to his arrested state of emotional development: an inverted baseball cap. Fortunately, this pop psychographic threatens neither social progress nor the present analysis.

Traditional team sports such as Baseball, Basketball and

Introduction

Football mirror traditional values: teamwork, cooperation, conformity, achievement, character-building, and healthy competition. Unlike traditional sports, the new genre of Extreme Sports, also dubbed "Millennial", "Alternative" or "Active Sports" (preferred by Generation Y) are solitary activities rooted in a diametrically opposite set of norms and characteristics that include fierce individualism, antisocial behavior, alienation, defiance, and most desperately -- a need to escape the lunacy of screaming coaches and frothing parents.

To the degree they exist, rabid parents and coaches do not have a place in a theory of humanistic evolution. But youth research conducted by American Sports Data, Inc. in 2001 suggests that this putative segment is small -- an overblown media trend, fueled by a tiny minority of adults responsible for uncommon incidents at Little League, Soccer or Hockey Games. Unfortunately, a rare episode of inter-parental violence easily captures the national spotlight.

In 2004, Team Sports were still the dominant form of Outdoors youth recreation, claiming 22 million frequent participants (25+ days per year), versus only 9.8 million for Extreme Sports. Overall, both sectors have been losing ground, consistent with declining athleticism, a childhood obesity epidemic, and other evidence -- anecdotal and empirical -- of a severe physical crisis among our nation's youth.

The new youth culture (now synonymous with Gen Y) has invaded dress, music, language, social interaction, sports spectatorship and the new "Alternative" sports. But while various features of the subculture appear woven into the social fabric, "Generation Y" is nothing more than a demographic category aspiring to psychographic status. In reality, Gen Y is a small slice of the much larger 6-24 age cohort, and this celebrated typology -- itself fragmented into Goth, Skater, Grunge, Surfer, Punk and Retro looks -- shares the limelight with other subcultures: Hip Hop, Preppy, Hipster and most ignored -- the dominant majority of "conventional" youngsters.

THE TWO FACES OF TECHNOLOGY

Since the industrial revolution, technology has been the natural enemy of physical activity. Indeed, the shift from agriculture to the new sedentary lifestyle in the big cities of Europe inspired one Hippolyte Triat in 1847 to open the first health club in Paris.

Workplace innovation, the automobile, telephone, television and the computer have been successive historical scapegoats for diminishing physical activity. Now, the gigantic lever of the Internet -- with email, surfing, chatrooms, instant messaging, music and video games -- has opened a huge chasm between outdoors and indoor recreation. There are other proofs, but the easiest evidence for this seismic shift is found in the decline of sports participation among 12-17 year-olds, a childhood obesity epidemic, vanishing PE programs and withering school athletics.

Introduction

And then there is the most terrifying prospect of all -- a competing scenario in which people never exercise. In this dystopian future, technology is finally triumphant, inventing a "magic pill" which supplies all nutriment, prevents weight gain, and otherwise ensures perfect health. Good news for pharmaceutical companies, but not necessarily for fitness.

On the other hand, the "natural enemy" metaphor is flawed because technology is also a friend, making more than ample restitution to Physical Fitness through interactive virtual reality, wireless electronic training aids, intelligent wristwatches and pedometers, remote heart rate sensors, the fusion of fitness and entertainment, and incipiently, a new era of digitized healthcare -- where both healthy and sick will be monitored, electronically prompted and medically treated from afar. Technology offers myriad unimagined blessings -- or their opposite -- for health and Physical Fitness.

WAVE OF THE FUTURE: SUBSIDIZED PHYSICAL FITNESS

For thousands of years, medicine has been "reactive"...it has been "remedial" and "curative". Therapeutic medicine has been the exclusive province of doctors who were summoned after-the-fact of disease, to treat sick or disabled people.

We are now on the threshold of yet another paradigm. Medical professionals and society in general have come to realize that keeping people healthy (preventive medicine) is far more economically sound than the old paradigm of treating them after-the-fact of illness, injury or disability (remedial medicine). HMO's, big business and government are finally -- but reluctantly -- acknowledging that healthier lifestyles translate into fewer HMO/PPO claims, higher workplace productivity, and fewer demands on an already strapped government healthcare system.

Under remedial healthcare, the doctor was the key player. In the new paradigm of preventive healthcare, the patient -- through self-monitoring and self-administration of a healthier lifestyle -- will assume the leading role. The trend toward healthier people through preventive healthcare will be subsidized by HMO's which are already issuing premium rebates for Health Club attendance and other healthy practices; by large employers who continue to build wellness centers; by Federal tax legislation, which has recently become amenable to fitness and Obesity-related tax deductions; by government policymakers on all levels, who as previously noted, have endorsed Obesity as a genuine "disease" -- worthy of Medicare benefits.

Americans regard healthcare as a basic necessity and right…with only a small step remaining to the subsidization of gym memberships, diet plans, nutritional supplements, and many other preventive healthcare measures. Physical Fitness will soon be a standard health benefit, even an entitlement. And this will have something to do with humanistic evolution.

* * *

PART ONE:

INTERVIEWS

Interviews

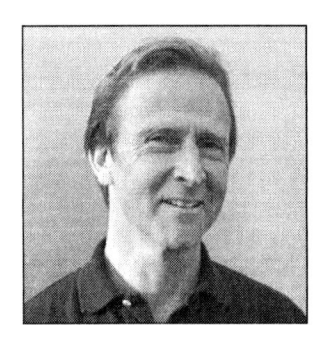

CHAPTER 1

THE LAUER REPORT: INSIGHTS FROM STATISTICS
by *Catherine Masterson McNeil*

For nearly two decades, Harvey Lauer, the president of American Sports Data, Inc. (ASD), a research firm based in Hartsdale, New York, has been tracking the statistics that tell the story of the American fitness movement. His persistent pursuit of the numbers, coupled with his knowledge of exercise and human psychology, has provided the fitness industry not only with facts, but also *enlightenment*.

"Physical exercise is inherently painful and inconvenient, and it defies the 'pleasure principle,'" he observes. "Some people may disagree with that notion, but the point is that most of us need some sort of external motivation to exercise. That's why health club memberships and personal training are growing, despite a stagnating fitness movement."

Still fit and trim at age 59, Lauer, a former sub-three-hour marathoner, understands, from his own experience, the value of group support. "I started running in the late 1970s because I was out of shape and overweight, and felt I just had to do something," he says. So Lauer joined, and eventually became president of, the Scarsdale (New York) Antiques, a running club founded by mature adults. "The group support really helped to get me going," he recalls.

At about the same time, Lauer began working for the Public Agenda Foundation, a public policy research organization, established in 1975, by statesman Cyrus Vance and social psychologist Daniel Yankelovich. Lauer had met the latter while pursuing a master's degree in psychology at the New School for Social Research in New York City, where Yankelovich was a visiting professor of psychology.

"As a $3-per-hour graduate student, I was the foundation's charter employee," muses Lauer. In 1983, Lauer seized the opportunity to integrate his two main passions -- running and research -- and launched the *Comprehensive Study of the American Runner*. Shortly thereafter, ASD was born.

Frequently referenced by the media, ASD conducts research that influences the fitness industry in both subtle and dramatic ways. Among the firm's more than 150 clients are: Coca-Cola; L.L. Bean; Sears; IHRSA, the Sporting Goods Manufacturers Association (SGMA); venture capital companies; fitness equipment manufacturers; health club chains; universities; and *USA Today, Reader's Digest*, and other major publications.

A highly disciplined man himself, Lauer has long struggled to understand why most Americans seem to lack the fortitude required to exercise regularly and achieve their fitness goals. His desire to make sense of that issue, and in some way, to have a positive impact on the population, has been at the heart of many of the studies he's undertaken.

Lauer employs two of his other passions—writing and rhetoric—to breathe life into the charts and graphs that constitute much of his work. Though adamant about being cautious when using research statistics, Lauer has a tendency to make use of colorful adjectives and a clever turn of phrase to drive home the meaning behind the numbers. Consider, for example, the following quote from one of his press releases -- or, as he calls them, "essays" -- regarding the need for a greater focus on youth fitness:

"Historically, teenagers have been powerful calorie-burning machines who -- though blasé about weight control and fitness until they grew older and heavier—naturally gravitated toward such youthful pursuits as baseball, skateboarding, basketball, volleyball, and hiking. But even here -- despite the growing popularity of 'extreme' sports, and evidence of increased health club usage due to the growth of family memberships -- overall participation numbers for the 12–17 age group are in severe decline. This not only represents a major assault on the sporting goods industry's bottom line, but is also a chilling omen for the future of public health in the U.S."

If we're to help ensure a healthier future for our nation's youth—i.e., tomorrow's health club members—it's important, concludes Lauer, that club operators make every effort to "raise the consciousness of educators, public offices, and, especially, parents—individuals who can make the most difference in the lives of children."

Will the industry meet the challenge?

Lauer, rest assured, will keep us all posted.

* * *

This article originally appeared in the August 2002 issue of Club Business International.
Catherine Masterson McNeil is a contributing editor for Club Business International and can be reached at cmm@ihrsa.org.

CHAPTER 2

> CBI INTERVIEW

August 2003

"We've sliced, diced, and trended the health club market in so many ways that I can't even remember them all."

HARVEY LAUER, THE MAN BEHIND
AMERICAN SPORTS DATA, INC.,
HAS THE STATS THAT DEFINE, GUIDE,
AND DRIVE OUR INDUSTRY

By Bradley A. Keeny

CBI: In your studies, you've noted that the number of frequent committed exercisers hasn't increased appreciably for years, and that, as a percentage of population, they've actually declined. What does that suggest?

HARVEY LAUER: Around 1990, the fitness movement reached a plateau, and we've been sitting on it ever since. The world operates in cycles, and progress with respect to any particular phenomenon is never a straight 45° uptrend. Reality is a jagged graph line, with untidy fits and starts, ups and downs.

CBI: You've also reported, however, that between 1990 and 2001, the number of health club members in the U.S. has shot from 20.7 million to 33.8 million, a dramatic 63% increase. How do you explain that?

HL: I've been saying for years that the fitness industry is shaped by a simple, but monumental, tenet -- the pleasure principle. Nearly all human behavior, in fact, is driven by our desire to avoid pain and maximize pleasure. While exercise offers intrinsic, undeniable, benefits, for most people, it is also inherently painful, boring, inconvenient, or otherwise unpleasant. In order to succeed at exercise, people require outside motivation, discipline, knowhow, and even a little handholding. They know it, and fitness professionals know it, and this is why health clubs and personal trainers have been able to thrive despite a lackluster fitness environment.

CBI: Have people's attitudes towards clubs changed significantly over the past 5-10 years? To what extent do you expect them to change during the coming decade?

HL: Some of the negative stereotypes haven't changed: "Clubs are overcrowded… Clubs are pick-up places… Salesmen are pushy," and so forth. Those things, unfortunately, haven't changed. But there are also positive perceptions that remain constant: "Clubs provide expertise and motivation that you can't obtain on your own… Clubs provide a valuable service to the community," etc. What is changing is the *unspoken* personal acceptance of clubs. This is reflected in silent attitudes, which hold something like, "A health club is a place for me… There are people here just like me… I could do that… This could work for me."

CBI: Your studies, among others, confirm that most peo-

ple now recognize the value of regular exercise, but most don't put that belief into practice. When, if at all, will we reach the turning point -- when Americans' attitudes about the value of exercise begin to coincide with their actual behavior?

HL: Behavior already coincides with attitudes -- but only to the tune of about 20% of the population. More than 80% of Americans are already persuaded that physical activity is very important, but only about 20% get enough exercise. It's a gradual evolutionary process. Maybe it'll take another 50 years… but it won't happen overnight, with the fall of an axe or the pushing of a button.

CBI: Is there any possibility that it will never happen? Given what seems to be a monumental shift towards obesity, is it conceivable that our standards about what is normal and acceptable will change? That 'heavy' will be in? That club members will become a distinct minority, a fitness elite?

HL: No. There are at least three competing scenarios, but I don't think any one will ever win the day. (1) There's the possibility that the pharmaceutical companies will develop a magic pill that prevents weight gain, addresses every health need, etc., and negates any reason to exercise. But that's an unrealistic scenario, because more and more people will exercise for the intrinsic rewards—to feel better afterward, to become stronger or more confident, to get in better shape, etc. (2) The "fat and fit philosophy" that's emerged recently isn't a threat because it still requires that the overweight person be fit. (3) Club members a new fitness elite? No way! Half of club members are what our segmentation studies refer to as Consciousness III, or "Uninitiated Believers" -- people who believe in fitness, but *still* don't get enough exercise.

CBI: Some of the most important insights provided by your studies have to do with those segments, the four different levels of 'fitness consciousness' that quantify people's readiness to exercise. Why is it important that clubs understand these stages?

HL: First, as you're aware, there's Consciousness I, or the 'Nonbelievers.' This prehistoric race constitutes only 2% of the population and will soon be extinct. Consciousness II, which we've labeled 'Indifferent,' accounts for 16%, and is a bit more evolved, but not by much. Neither group is important in terms of the marketing of fitness-related products.

Consciousness III, representing 63%, is clearly the most important marketing target for clubs. These 'Uninitiated Believers' are already convinced of the virtues of fitness, and are ready to join, but many feel that they're unhealthy, overweight, and/or unathletic, and may be self-conscious about their bodies. They need to be lured with marketing strategies that are built around these psychographics.

Consciousness IV is the 'Hard-Core' fitness participant,

who makes up 17% of the population. Many of them are already club customers, and many others are committed to nonclub fitness activities, and not easily induced to switch to a club membership.

CBI: One of your fans has observed that this segmentation 'has clear implications in terms of where the low-hanging fruit for our industry is with respect to new members.'

HL: 'Low-hanging fruit' is an outstanding metaphor. From the perspective of our psychographic segmentation, Consciousness III, or the 'Uninitiated Believers,' represent the low-hanging fruit -- ripe and easy picking! At 128 million strong, they're by far the largest marketing target, and 73 million don't have a club affiliation or a fitness interest that would compete with belonging to a club.

Again, Consciousness IV is the 'Hard-Core' fitness participant, but most of this fruit has already been harvested, and the remainder hangs a lot higher in the tree -- some of it out of reach. This is because 63% are already club patrons or members, and 26% are frequent fitness participants who are committed to exercising out-of-doors or at home. It's probably not wise to try to convert people of other faiths.

Another example of low-hanging fruit is the huge number of nonmember patrons, a group that now includes about 25 million. These club users don't have memberships, but pay a daily fee, purchase a particular program, or make use of some other nondues arrangement, and, because of their current club experience, present a very high conversion potential.

CBI: If Consciousness III is, in fact, the most promising growth segment, what would you suggest that clubs do to reach them effectively?

HL: If you want to recruit Consciousness III, don't focus on conversion; in spirit, these people are already in the fold. Their attitudes have already changed, and all we have to do is help them change their behavior. Focus on everyday operational incentives, particularly less threatening exercise environments -- for instance, dress codes, same-gender facilities, mirrorless settings, less demanding forms of exercise, user-friendly equipment, fitness pampering, and special handholding. It also wouldn't hurt to tell them that, in conjunction with reasonable eating and other healthy habits, exercise really works.

CBI: Your newest report, *A Comprehensive Study of American Attitudes Toward Fitness and Health Clubs*, notes that nearly nine out of every 10 Americans now believe that regular exercise is essential to weight management. Is this realization making a difference?

HL: Absolutely. People have become less enchanted with dieting as a way to lose weight because it's not a permanent remedy. I think they're also becoming less enamored of diet pills, appetite suppressants, and other passive forms of weight control. If 88% of Americans believe that "regular exercise is essential to weight management" -- that says it all.

CBI: However, as you point out, health clubs are the fourth-most-popular way to lose weight, with 22 million adult participants, trailing far behind better eating habits (100 million), outdoor exercise (48 million), and home exercise (47 million). Why aren't clubs at the top of the list?

HL: You're right. Of the 59 million health club patrons -- both members and nonmembers -- only about 22 million utilize clubs to lose weight. Weight loss isn't the principal motive for purchasing a club membership. What clubs can do to improve their ranking is to emphasize that working out in a health club is the most effective way to lose weight -- a fact that's been documented, for the first time ever, in this new research. They should also stress the fact that the superior results provided by a club far outweigh the perceived inconvenience and imagined higher costs involved when compared with other exercise regimens.

CBI: The industry goal of 50 million members in the U.S. by 2010 is one that some observers regard as inevitable without any major changes or initiatives, but that others regard as challenging. What's your view?

HL: Achieving 50 million members by 2010 requires only a compound annual growth rate of 4%-5% for the next seven years. Many say it will be a walkthrough… but when it comes to betting on a sure thing, I like to keep my money in my pocket.

CBI: Okay, so you're not a betting man, but what advice would you offer the club industry about how to achieve 50 million members by 2010?

HL: I think what would easily put them over the top is a unified industry campaign that speaks with a single voice. Not one that preaches to the choir about the virtues of physical fitness, because your prospects are already believers, but, rather, a powerful series of messages that emphasize the functional, pragmatic, aspects of the club experience -- aimed squarely at Consciousness III. They're nearly ready to take the plunge, but many are still a little bit nervous about the details. Your advertising and marketing messages should stress that clubs are fun places, with light weights, user-friendly equipment, and weight-loss classes, where they'll meet people just like themselves. From an operational point of view, clubs should cater to an older population by providing an older staff, appropriate equipment, relevant classes, such as mind/body and weight control, and less taxing programs, such as Yoga and Pilates. But, at the same time, don't forget your roots -- the traditional health club member; the 18-34-year-old hardbody still constitutes 36% of the commercial club population.

CBI: Industry leaders are constantly talking about the 13%-14% of the population that belongs to clubs, sug-

gesting that they regard the other 86%-87% as prospects. How realistic a notion is that? What would a realistic penetration rate for the U.S. be?

HL: Good question. I certainly don't think that the reciprocal 86% of nonmembers represents a realistic universe of prospects. Here's a seat-of-the-pants estimate: There are 207 million adults in the U.S. Let's guess that 30 million are very old, disabled, or otherwise incapable of much in the way of physical activity. Let's also guess that, at the moment, another 50 million are incorrigible couch potatoes, even though some of them may be Consciousness III. Another 35 million may be frequent exercisers who don't utilize a club, and over 30 million are already club members. That would leave around 60 million, or 30%-35% of the adult population, as a more reasonable universe of prospects.

CBI: We noticed that your client list doesn't include many club companies. How can club owners do a better job of mining and leveraging the sort of statistical information that you provide?

HL: The *Comprehensive Study*, the report that we've been talking about here, is probably the most 'actionable' research report we've ever produced. In order to sell products in any market, you need to define that market -- demographically, geographically, psychographically, and by other methods of segmentation. We've sliced, diced, and trended the health club market in so many ways that I can't even remember them all. The immediate future of the health club industry is Consciousness III -- anyone who's involved in this business needs to know who these people are and what they're thinking. Because of this particular report, for instance, club owners can now advertise -- with confidence and scientific support -- that club members are more successful than nonmembers with their weight-loss efforts. For the first time ever, ASD has proved it. That's huge!

CBI: If you were to plot the principal metrics that you follow for health clubs for, say, the next 10 years, what would we see -- in terms of number of clubs, total number of members, number of frequent exercisers, etc.?

HL: As a charter member, in 1967, of the World Future Society, I was once very interested in futuristic prediction: I was fond of saying that the long-range future is easier to forecast than the near-term. My standard prophecy: "In the fitness utopia of 2050, every able-bodied American works out every day; and those who don't are social outcasts -- like the rare misfits who didn't brush their teeth every day back in 2003." Over the next 5-10 years? Well, that's a little more difficult. As I said before, I'll keep my money in my pocket.

* * *

BRADLEY A. KEENY *is the associate editor of CBI and can be reached at b.keeny@fit-etc.com.*

Interviews

CHAPTER 3

HEALTH & FITNESS BUSINESS
(An Interview with Harvey Lauer -- July 2004)

JULY 01, 2004 — Want to know what the American fitness consumer is thinking? Ask Harvey Lauer, president of American Sports Data, Inc. For the past 19 years, ASD has been the specialist in consumer research for the sporting goods, fitness and health club industries. ASD is the principal provider of consumer research for both the Sporting Goods Manufacturers Association (SGMA) and the International Health & Racquet Sportsclub Association (IHRSA).

Lauer is known for his precise research and plainly spoken opinions. Here are the highlights of a recent conversation with SGB's Health & Fitness Business.

H&FB: As an industry expert, how do you regard today's consumers? What are they doing, and how are they spending their money?

LAUER: Thank you for the elevation to "expert", but that's true only in the narrow sense of national consumer research. Since I usually don't fly that low, I can't say what's going on inside the retail trenches. But here's the view from 10,000 feet. Physical fitness today is simplicity itself. The vast majority of the population (over 80%)

believes in fitness; but only 20% gets enough exercise. People have difficulty with self-motivation. That's why, over the last decade, home exercise has been flat, while health clubs -- and until recently the personal trainer business -- has been booming! People, simply can't do it on their own. They need help.

But if they must do it on their own, fitness consumers need "easy" exercise equipment. This is why light hand weights, recumbent bikes and yoga have become so popular. Second, they need external motivation, somehow piped into the home -- special videos, email encouragement, Internet personal training or other applications and incentives we haven't even dreamed of. And then there's the issue of tangible and attainable fitness goals. I think this is a propitious time for intelligent pedometers, heart rate monitors, body measurement and fitness tracking devices. When people have clearly defined goals that they're often reminded of, they'll stick with exercise and weight control a lot longer.

H&FB: What are the differences between the health club consumer and the home fitness consumer?

LAUER: Home exercisers lack the external incentives provided by a health club environment -- social interaction, peer pressure, expertise, and discipline, to name a few. But these are motivational techniques and devices that can be imported into the home. Some of these ideas are "futuristic", some are already on the horizon, and a few have been around for a while. I'm talking about motivational videos, "remote" personal training, exercise buddies in chat rooms, regular inspirational emails to bolster morale, new tracking and monitoring technology, economic incentives, the weight watcher's concept somehow imported into the home, and still other unforeseen motivational strategies.

If you want to analyze the differences between these two groups, right now, frequent health club users are more "masculine", younger and more affluent than frequent home exercisers. 52% of frequent health club attendees are male, versus 45% of frequent home exercisers. 56% of these frequent club users are over 35, compared with 64% for the home fitness crowd. And not surprisingly, nearly half -- 48% of frequent club patrons -- have incomes above $75,000, as opposed to a still-respectable 40% of all frequent home exercisers.

H&FB: How is the situation different from five years ago?

LAUER: The situation differs from five years ago in that things are reaching a boiling point. The ASD Superstudy® of Sports Participation now measures weight, height and body mass index...and guess what? The average adult female weighs in at over 160 lbs, while men tip the scales at over 190! These alarming numbers are confirmed by CDC research. American eating behavior is on a rampage, while physical activity levels have remained stagnant or have declined -- so only one result is possible: an explosion of the national waistline! Now, things are coming to a head. People have been fitness-conscious for years, but the public is now being rocked by a tremendous amount of publicity and buzz about a full-blown obesity epidemic...with daily newspaper coverage of unacceptable collateral damage -- diabetes, heart disease, and other life-threatening risks. Big Food companies are on the bandwagon with radical reforms in fat content, portion sizes and major overhauling of school cafeterias. HMO's and insurance companies are issuing premium rebates for health club attendance, and the IRS may be five years away from allowing 1040 deductions for healthy lifestyle expenditures. So all this commotion is starting to move the needle. My latest numbers reflect a little bump in fitness participation -- over and above soaring health club memberships.

H&FB: What are your impressions of young fitness consumers?

LAUER: In my opinion, today's kids are the most spoiled generation in American history -- regardless of socioeconomic status. Few have experienced need or deprivation, while parents, grandparents, advertisers and other guilty parties have nurtured excessive expectations. They're also less connected to fitness than kids of previous generations, and their renunciation of physical activity is already a cliché. It's blamed on lots of things, but most notably a seismic shift from outdoor to indoor recreation. The usual, guilty suspects are email, chat rooms, Internet surfing, video games, music and other new indoor distractions. Vanishing PE programs, withering school sports, the disappearance of pickup games are other culprits. The so-called Extreme Sports -- despite all the hype and hoopla -- have not taken up the slack, certainly not in terms of total participation and caloric expenditure. Naturally, the most glaring symptom of youthful inactivity is the much-publicized childhood obesity epidemic.

If kids were interested in fitness, they would spend money on it. It seems that social class or a low household income are not obstacles to a slew of "new necessities", which in any other era, would have been luxuries. Most kids have cell phones, video games, loads of CD's, designer clothing, travel sports teams, and spring break in Myrtle Beach or Cancun. Kids of my generation -- even those better placed in the social order -- were lucky to get near the Catskills in a crammed, broken-down family car!

This situation is lopsided and counterintuitive, but it's true because of vast changes in our culture, lifestyles, demographics and most of all -- a new "juvenile psychology of entitlement". In the Inner City, we often find both parents of a marginal household holding two, even three jobs; and in blue-collar, Lower Middle America, long-ravaged by outsourcing and other economic decay, a demanding child has four live grandparents (they live longer today) to help with these "necessities". All this amidst a widening gap between rich and poor...

We can attack the problem on several fronts. We need more evangelism like Jim Baugh's P.E.4Life, more kids programs at health clubs, health initiatives to persuade both parents and educators that inactivity literally <u>kills</u> children. And most of all, we need fitness-minded parental role models -- the only people that will make a difference.

H&FB: What about the 50-plus crowd?

LAUER: I can relate to the over-50 crowd, and that's a much better story. Seniors are actually propping up the fitness movement; and this is a trend no one saw coming. Since 1987 for example, health club membership is up 127%; but for people 55+, the number is +343%! From 1998 - 2003, Pilates is the number one growth activity (+445%), followed by Yoga/Tai Chi (+134%). Both are predominantly female, and skewed "older" than the general fitness population. Recumbent Cycling, the second "oldest" activity measured, has increased by 58% during the same period.

There are several reasons for the graying of the fitness boom -- if we can call it that. One is that there are many fitness participants like me -- people who started running in the late 1970's, and maintained the fitness lifestyle. Forty year-olds in 1980 became sixty year-olds in 2000...

Another reason for the popularity of senior fitness is that it's now socially acceptable...When we were kids growing up in the Bronx, if my mother looked out the window and saw an old man running around in his underwear, she would have called the police!

A third reason is therapeutic referral; huge numbers of medical professionals are prescribing physical activity as an antidote to osteoporosis, heart disease, diabetes and a host of other maladies. Still another explanation for the aging fitness boom is that equipment manufacturers have accommodated older folks with user-friendly equipment for Kinder/Gentler fitness...The context was more general, but my favorite slide in the ASD Health & Fitness Expo presentation last year was "Make It Easy and They Will Come".

H&FB: Why are you bullish on the future of fitness?

LAUER: I'm bullish on the future of fitness because I believe in what I'm fond of calling the "inexorable march of humanistic evolution". Although sociological arguments can be made to the contrary, I think that people are becoming smarter and more sensitive about their planet, their environment, their relationships with other people, and also their bodies. Right now we're on the threshold of a great leap forward in physical fitness -- but not necessarily because of philosophical enlightenment. It's because enough people and enough institutions now realize that physical inactivity is becoming dangerous to our collective health.

* * *

PART TWO:

PHYSICAL FITNESS

CHAPTER 4

GRANDPARENTS FITTER THAN GRANDCHILDREN?

FOR IMMEDIATE RELEASE   July 23, 2001

* * *

National Tracking Study Reveals Startling Role Reversal: Seniors Over 55 Exercise More Frequently Than Any Age Group -- Especially Teenagers

* * *

Vanishing Phys Ed Programs and Sedentary Distractions Fuel a Growing National Obesity Crisis Among Children

HARTSDALE, N.Y. -- Nearly 1 out of 4 health club members in the U.S. (23%) are now at least 55 years old. This growing army of 7.3 million older fitness enthusiasts has mushroomed by 379% since 1987 -- four times as fast as the general health club population. These were among the findings of the 14th annual Superstudy® of Sports Participation, conducted in January 2001 by American Sports Data, Inc.

Counting all forms of exercise, including gym workouts, 26% of all seniors over the age of 55 participated in a single fitness activity on at least 100 occasions -- the highest incidence for any age group. This compares with 23% for the 35-54 age category, 20% for those 18-34 and only 18% of children aged 12-17 who were frequent fitness participants in the year 2000 -- "a dangerous decline from the rate of 31% measured for teens in 1987," according to ASD president Harvey Lauer.

Historically, teenagers have been powerful calorie-burning machines who -- though blasé about weight control and fitness until they grew older and heavier -- naturally gravitated toward such youthful pursuits as baseball, skateboarding, basketball, volleyball and hiking. But even here -- despite the growing popularity of "Extreme" sports and evidence of increased health club usage due to the growth of family memberships -- overall participation numbers for the 12-17 age group are in severe decline. "This", says Lauer, "represents not only a major assault on the sporting goods industry's bottom line, but is also a chilling omen for the future of public health in the U.S."

According to the Centers for Disease Control, daily participation in high school physical education classes has fallen dramatically - from 42% in 1991 to 27% in 1997. More than 1 out of 5 adolescents in the U.S. are overweight; 14% are classified as obese. Both measurements have risen precipitously from CDC reports in the 1980's.

Explanations abound for the demise of teen activity. In addition to the disappearance of Physical Education, the usual suspects are web surfing, e-mail, chat rooms, Nintendo, video games, CD's, MTV, piano lessons, SAT coaching, Girls Scout meetings and a host of other frenetic but sedentary distractions that fill the life of the "overscheduled" child at the turn of the Millennium. There may have been a seismic shift in the venue of youthful recreation from outdoors to indoors, but some things never change. The voracious time culprit -- according to a 1999 study by the Kaiser Foundation -- is still television, not the computer. Children aged 2-18 spend an average of 2 hours 46 minutes per day watching TV, compared with only 8 minutes on the Internet, and 20 minutes playing computer games. Kids spend an additional 21 minutes on the computer for 'fun'.

If present trends continue at both ends of the age spectrum, will this fitness paradox culminate in 60 year-olds outrunning 16 year-olds? Technically, the 55+ age group is the most fitness-conscious demographic in America -- but this doesn't imply that seniors exercise with an intensity equal to that of their children or grandchildren. Older people adopt fitness programs consonant with their capabilities: fitness walking, stationary cycling, stretching, treadmill exercise and hand weights are among the most popular. There are many exceptions, but potentially more strenuous activities such as running, high-impact aerobics or barbells are skewed much younger.

The willingness to exercise is far more important than the content or format of the activity. "The important thing", Lauer adds, "is that people do whatever their bodies will allow. That 26% of all seniors exercise frequently is even more amazing, when you consider that for reasons of infirmity, disability or very old age, a good number of older people may be incapable of physical activity."

Other ASD research has consistently demonstrated that most Americans are sold on the idea of fitness -- but this has only created a yawning chasm that separates positive attitudes from actual fitness behavior. "Not too many people argue with the wisdom of fitness", said Lauer. "Over 80% of the population endorses the concept of physical activity for better health, but only 20% gets nearly enough exercise."

Why have seniors, more than any other age group, been able to make the leap from this highly developed fitness-consciousness to actual fitness behavior? The prosaic explanation is that they simply have more time; but because this has always been true, it is the least compelling interpretation. A more cogent reason according to ASD, is that many were recruited during the early stages of the fitness boom, and are just graduating to the top age bracket. When compared with a generation ago, exercise is far more often mandated by a doctor, physical therapist or other medical health professional. And for most, preventive health concerns become more immediate with age, as the confrontation with one's mortality begins to inspire all manner of life-prolonging activity.

Beneath the loftier motivational analyses lie the simpler but perhaps not-so-obvious realities: mirroring the evolution of female fitness, vigorous activity in one's twilight years is now socially acceptable -- not embarrassing. But most important, seniors now believe they are capable of exercise -- thanks in part to an accommodating fitness industry.

Indeed, most of the recent growth in physical fitness has been of the "kinder and gentler" low-impact or no-impact variety, crediting its success to an influx of older converts. From 1998 - 2000, participation gains have been recorded in Recumbent Cycling (+32%); Yoga/Tai Chi (+30%); Hand Weights (+16%); and Treadmill Exercise (+10%). In a first-time-ever measurement, Pilates Training registered 1.7 million participants, 60% of whom were first-year entrants in 2000.

How can our fitness-challenged, if not "endangered", youngsters benefit from the wisdom of their elders? It's probably too much of a stretch to imagine they can, concludes Lauer. "The mature market has some compelling exercise incentives that are unique to that group. For kids, the bottom line is to raise the consciousness of educators, public officials and especially parents -- the influentials who can make the most difference in the lives of children."

The Superstudy® of Sports Participation was conducted in January 2001 and based on a nationally representative sample of 14,772 people over the age of 6, who were among 25,000 respondents targeted in a sample drawn from the consumer mail panel of NFO Research, Inc. 103 sports and activities were measured along 20 demographic, attitudinal and behavioral dimensions. Data were also collected on health club membership and other subjects pertinent to physical fitness. This annual tracking study has been conducted by ASD every year since 1987, and sponsored by the Sporting Goods Manufacturers Association of North Palm Beach, Florida. For more information, log onto www.americansportsdata.com.

* * *

SELECTED ACTIVITY PARTICIPATION*
AGE 12 - 17 (Per 100 People)

	1987	1993	2000
Baseball	26.5	22.7	11.5
Basketball	54.8	57.4	45.5
Football (Touch)	35.5	33.4	22.6
Free Weights	25.1	28.5	27.1
In-Line Skating	n.a.	16.9	30.3
Running/Jogging	42.6	37.9	31.2
Skateboarding	21.3	8.4	16.8
Soccer	29.4	25.1	20.7
Softball	36.6	33.1	16.1
Snowboarding	n.a.	4.5	9.1
Tennis	23.7	20.7	13.3
Volleyball	48.9	46.3	26.0
Weight/Resistance Machines	9.6	6.9	13.1

*at least once per year
Source: American Sports Data, Inc.

Grandparents Fitter than Grandchildren?

SELECTED ACTIVITY PARTICIPATION*
AGE 55+ (Per 100 People)

	1987	1993	2000
Aerobics	2.5	2.8	4.7
Fitness Walking	15.9	18.3	20.2
Free Weights	1.6	2.3	11.2
Running/Jogging	2.7	1.8	3.8
Stationary Cycling	11.1	12.3	12.2
Stair-Climbers	.3	2.6	3.7
Treadmill Exercise	1.8	6.7	17.3
Weight/Resistance Machines	1.7	2.2	7.2

*at least once per year
Source: American Sports Data, Inc.

* * *

CHAPTER 5

NATIONAL TRACKING STUDY IDENTIFIES NEW FITNESS MANTRAS: FLEXIBILITY AND STRENGTH TRAINING

FOR IMMEDIATE RELEASE   April 25, 2002

* * *

Pilates, Elliptical Trainers, Yoga, Hand Weights and Other User-Friendly Activities Supplement Traditional 1990's Cardio Exercise

* * *

But Losses in Other Activities Slows Overall Fitness Growth to a Standstill

HARTSDALE, N.Y. -- Cardiovascular exercise, centerpiece of the 1980's and 1990's fitness culture, is being heavily reinforced by two other essential pillars of physical health -- flexibility and strength-training. From 1998-2001, aggregate participation in Cardio workouts has been statistically flat (-2%), lagging far behind the growth of Strength-Training (+12%) and Flexibility/Stretching activities, which have flared by +23%. These were among the findings of the 15th annual Superstudy® of Sports Participation, conducted in January 2002 among 14,276 Americans nationwide by American Sports Data, Inc. (ASD).

Accommodating legions of women, older enthusiasts and deconditioned beginners, the fastest growing exercise forms tend to be workouts that are less taxing or take a lesser toll on the body -- and at the same time, help provide a balanced fitness regimen.

The top growth activity was Pilates Training, which increased to 2.4 million participants in 2001 -- a 40% leap over the initial year 2000 measurement of 1.7 million. This hybrid endeavor (a blend of stretching, balance and strength exercise) is dominated by women, who constitute 85% of all participants. Elliptical Motion Trainers -- "no-impact" pedaling machines that are particularly amenable to those with knee problems -- surged by 34% in the past year and by 114% since 1998. The compound measurement of Yoga/Tai Chi yielded 9.7 million adherents in 2001 -- up from 6.2 million in 2000 (+32%) and 5.7 million in 1998 (+71%).

While the activity of Stretching has grown from 35.1 million participants in 1998 to 38.1 million in 2001 (an increase of 9%) its relatively youthful demographics (average age 34.7) are suggestive of ancillary warm-ups and warm-downs -- serving a main sport or fitness activity. But for many people, especially those over the age of 55 (who constitute 19% of this population), Stretching is an important exercise in its own right.

The analysis of Strength Training is far more complex, according to ASD president Harvey Lauer. "One reason for the growth of this component," he states, "is the general elevation of fitness in the public mind, and our realization that strength is an essential ingredient of health. But just as important, the evolution of social values is <u>allowing</u> women and older exercisers to participate without stigma or self-consciousness. And the third thing is that by ingeniously providing user-friendly products and actively promoting a new brand of low-stress fitness -- the industry is <u>enabling</u> these groups to participate."

In the 1950's and even the 1960's, weight lifting was not a socially acceptable activity for women. But in 2001, women accounted for 45% of all those who train with Free Weights, up from the ASD benchmark measurement of 30% in 1987. Of all people who use Hand Weights of five pounds or less, women comprise a 60% majority.

In a fascinating parallel to the history of female fitness, vigorous activity in one's twilight years is no longer an embarrassment -- or worse, a vaguely deviant behavior. In 2001, 13% of all Free Weights users were aged 55+, compared with only 3% in 1987.

Aquatic Exercise, another user-friendly activity, claimed 7.1 million adherents in 2001, a jump of 12% from the previous year. This kinder, and arguably gentlest of all fitness pursuits is dominated by women (77%) and represented by the second largest percentage of seniors over 55 (24%) for any fitness endeavor. With 27% of its participants over the age of 55, only Fitness Walking surpasses Aquatic Exercise in the advanced age of its constituency.

A kindred exercise, Fitness Swimming, reflected a 9% gain in 2001. With a population of 36.4 million, Fitness Walking has maintained an even keel in recent years; and to the surprise of some, middle age has not totally decimated the ranks of its younger sibling activity -- Running/Jogging, which claims 34.9 million participants. Compared with 1998, the Running/Jogging population remains unchanged; but it is 4% higher than the year 2000 measurement.

While many fitness activities are edging upward, others are moving south: Over the past three years, the biggest losers have been Aerobic Riders and Nordic Ski Machines -- infomercial-driven products whose usage has declined by 33% and 28% respectively. To the consternation of some observers, Outdoor Fitness Bicycling is also hemorrhaging, incurring a 21% loss in participants from 1998 - 2001. Stair-Climber usage and Aerobics have each suffered 19% declines during the same period, while another of yesterday's stars -- Cardio Kickboxing -- has endured a 12% participation loss from 1999 - 2001.

In the final analysis, says Lauer, "competing undercurrents are canceling out one another, giving the appearance of a relatively placid overall surface measurement of physical fitness." In 2001, 50.6 million people exercised at least 100 times in any single fitness activity, down from 51.7 million a year ago, and from 51.3 million in 1998.

Health club membership by contrast, grew from 32.8 million in 2000 to 33.8 million in 2001, a statistically insignificant gain of 3%. However, there has been a 7% increase over the past year in the number of health club patrons, who were not necessarily members. Since 1998, actual club membership has grown by 15%. The paradox of a robust health club industry in the face of a stagnating fitness movement can be explained, according to Lauer, as the sum of several factors: a raised level of health and fitness consciousness among Americans; the recognition of many would-be fitness participants that they need an external source of motivation; and despite a considerable rate of turnover -- the ability of health clubs to retain active members. In 2001, health club members in the U.S. logged an aggregate of 3.1 billion visits, an increase of 25% over 1998.

The Superstudy® of Sports Participation was conducted in January 2002 and based on a nationally representative sample of 14,276 people over the age of 6, who were among 25,000 respondents targeted in a sample drawn from the consumer mail panel of NFO Research, Inc. 103 sports and activities were measured along over 20 demographic, attitudinal and behavioral dimensions. Data were also collected on health club membership and other subjects pertinent to physical fitness. This annual tracking study has been conducted by ASD every year since 1987, and sponsored by the Sporting Goods Manufacturers Association of North Palm Beach, Florida. For more information, log onto www.americansportsdata.com.

SELECTED FITNESS ACTIVITIES
Participated at least once (000)
1998-2001

	1998	1999	2000	2001	1-Year Change 2000-2001	3-Year Change 1998-2001
Pilates Training	n.a.	n.a.	1,739	2,437	+40%	n.a.
Elliptical Motion Trainers	3,863	5,081	6,176	8,255	+34%	+114%
Yoga/Tai Chi	5,708	6,404	7,400	9,741	+32%	+71%
Hand Weights	23,325	25,862	27,086	27,078	0	+16%
Weight/Resistance Machines	22,519	22,961	25,182	25,942	+3%	+15%
Dumbbells	23,414	24,754	25,241	26,773	+6%	+14%
Ab Machine/Device	16,534	17,109	18,119	18,692	+3%	+13%
Treadmill Exercise	37,073	37,463	40,816	41,638	+2%	+12%
Home Gym Exercise	7,577	7,918	8,103	8,497	+5%	+12%
Stretching	35,114	35,278	36,408	38,120	+5%	+9%
Barbells	21,263	21,717	21,972	23,030	+5%	+8%
Aquatic Exercise	6,685	5,557	6,367	7,103	+12%	+6%

SOURCE: AMERICAN SPORTS DATA, INC.

SELECTED FITNESS ACTIVITIES (Continued)
Participated at least once (000)
1998-2001

	1998	1999	2000	2001	1-Year Change 2000-2001	3-Year Change 1998-2001
Swimming (Laps/Fitness)	15,258	14,194	14,060	15,300	+ 9%	0
Running/Jogging	34,962	34,047	33,680	34,857	+ 4%	0
Fitness Walking	36,395	35,976	36,207	36,445	+ 1%	0
Stationary Cycling (Net)	30,791	30,942	28,795	28,720	0	- 7%
Cardio Kickboxing	n.a.	7,607	7,163	6,665	- 7%	- 12% [1]
Aerobics (Net)	21,017	19,129	17,326	16,948	- 2%	- 19%
Stair Climbers	18,609	16,288	15,828	15,117	- 5%	- 19%
Fitness Biking (Outdoors)	13,556	12,307	11,435	10,761	- 6%	- 21%
X-C Ski Machines	6,870	5,921	5,444	4,924	-10%	- 28%
Aerobic Riders	5,868	4,165	3,817	3,918	+ 3%	- 33%

(1) 2-year Change

SOURCE: AMERICAN SPORTS DATA, INC.

CHAPTER 6

THE GAP BETWEEN ATTITUDES AND BEHAVIOR: FOUR LEVELS OF FITNESS CONSCIOUSNESS

A near-unanimity of Americans (97%) regard good physical health as an important value; as a corollary, few aspects of American culture can match the weighty consensus enjoyed by the fitness phenomenon. Surveys conducted by American Sports Data, Inc. in 1996, 1998 and 2002 have replicated to within a percentage point that the vast majority of Americans (85%) acknowledge the importance of getting enough exercise.

But while the health and fitness movement has clearly won the hearts and minds of Americans, it has just begun to move the behavioral needle. In general, actual fitness participation does not even begin to approach enlightened attitudes. While the numbers are inching upward, in 2002, only a sixth of the adult population (17%) could be classified as hard-core participants who -- in addition to extolling the virtues of physical activity -- are also avid practitioners.

To the endless delight of the fitness industry and media, I am fond of repeating that behavior simply lags good intentions; that people are truly becoming smarter about their bodies and that "humanistic evolution" will ultimately win the day; and that by the year 2050, all able-bodied people will exercise. Those who do not will be outcasts -- held in the same esteem as those who did not brush their teeth every day back in 2003.

On the other hand, technology and scientific advancement -- the natural enemies of physical activity -- could also win the day. Indeed, 38% of the adult population stated in 2002 that if a "magic pill" were available, they would cut back exercise.

Another formidable adversary of fitness is the "Pleasure Principle". In its true incarnation, this is something more complex; but in common parlance, the Pleasure Principle refers simply to the seeking of pleasure and the avoidance of pain. Exercise is time-consuming, inconvenient, even painful; and while it offers certain pleasures, attractions, is said even to cause addictions, on balance -- it is rife with motivational obstacles. At this evolutionary stage, strenuous physical activity is avoided by most Americans. Small wonder that health clubs and personal trainers (benefiting from a massive failure of self-motivation) have flourished in an environment of stagnating fitness behavior. In 1990, there were 51.5 million people in the U.S. aged 6+ who participated at least 100 times in a single fitness activity. Eleven years later, in 2001 -- even with population expansion -- the number had stalled at 50.6 million. During the same period, the number of health club members soared by 63%.

The following segmentation demonstrates our perennial lack of self-discipline; Americans know they can't do it on their own, and are primed to receive even more help from health clubs, personal trainers and the nascent phenomenon of incentivized physical fitness. Consciousness III (Uninitiated Believers) represents 63% of the population -- a colossal opportunity for the health and fitness industry.

Four Levels of Fitness Consciousness

AN "A PRIORI" FITNESS SEGMENTATION OF THE U.S. POPULATION

This segmentation of the U.S. population was <u>not</u> derived from multivariate statistical analysis; it is simply a single question which requires the respondent to self-select one of four typologies.

The most "evolved" segment of the population is designated Consciousness IV -- "hard-core" fitness enthusiasts who comprise 17% of the population.

But the dominant segment is a huge untapped market -- the army of "Uninitiated Believers" who need only make the leap from receptive attitudes to actual behavior. This "silent" majority (Consciousness III) comprises 63% of the population, and is the future of fitness.

While somewhat open-minded about the value of exercise and healthy lifestyles, a small minority of Americans (dubbed "Indifferent") disclaim a personal interest in physical fitness. These Consciousness II personalities (16% of the population) are not likely converts.

At the lowest rung of the fitness hierarchy is the tiny, antiquated (and probably vanishing) breed of "Non-Believers", who are least amenable (if not downright inimical!) to the idea of physical fitness. Facing extinction, the Consciousness I segment comprises only 2% of the adult population.

While the contingent of hard-core participants appeared to edge upward, from 1996 - 2002 there were no statistically significant changes in any of the four levels of Fitness Consciousness.

LEVELS OF FITNESS CONSCIOUSNESS

	1996 %	1998 %	2002 %
I NON-BELIEVERS "I just don't think exercise is all that important."	2	2	2
II INDIFFERENT "Exercise may be important, but I just don't feel the need to get involved in fitness activities."	17	18	16
III UNINITIATED BELIEVERS "I know exercise is important, and I'd like to participate in fitness activities more than I do."	64	62	63
IV HARD-CORE PARTICIPANTS "Exercise is very important to me, and I am a frequent participant in fitness activities"	15	16	17
Not Reported	2	2	2
	100	100	100

"NON-BELIEVERS" -- CONSCIOUSNESS I

This "Non-Believer" group is the least "enlightened" of the four fitness typologies. Dominated by men, this segment is the oldest and least educated.

Members of this rare species are more likely to smoke, and also less likely to watch their diets. While the sub-sample is very small, a large majority (74%) can be safely classified as sedentary.

When compared with the general population, this "old world" group is not especially overweight; but neither does it profess good health. This vanishing enclave is least receptive to the idea of exercise and fitness, and does not embrace the fitness lifestyle -- in either word or deed. A substantial number say that they are confused about whether exercise is really good or bad, while 60% believe that with good nutrition and a clean life, exercise really isn't necessary.

Consciousness I occupies the lowest rung of a 20th century Maslovian hierarchy. This primitive breed is stuck in mid-century, unaware of self-fulfillment, preventive healthcare and even the ego-driven motivation for physical self-enhancement. These ideas belong to a more evolved future.

This "Non-Believer" group continues to represent only 2% of the study sample.

"INDIFFERENT" -- CONSCIOUSNESS II

Consciousness II individuals are higher on the evolutionary scale, but not by much. Compared with Non-Believers they are somewhat more open-minded and receptive to the idea of exercise, but they too disavow a personal interest in physical fitness.

Consciousness II is equally divided by gender, and is of low income and education. Nearly 6 out of 10 (57%) fall into the sedentary category.

In general, this group has fairly negative attitudes about fitness, but not to the extreme of Consciousness I; but compared with those of more highly developed levels of consciousness (III & IV) this group is less concerned about diet and are far more likely to smoke cigarettes. They are far less active than these more fitness-conscious groups, and also far less prone to claim excellent health than are hard-core enthusiasts. Somewhat ironically, when compared with Consciousness III, this "Indifferent" segment is somewhat less likely to be overweight -- and equally healthy.

Consciousness II accounted for 16% of the study sample.

"UNINITIATED BELIEVERS" -- CONSCIOUSNESS III

Members of this group believe in the values and benefits of fitness, but for a variety of reasons, are unable to translate attitude into action. 25% are totally sedentary, while 26% of the Consciousness III group are already active sports/fitness participants (150+ days per year) who admonish themselves for not doing even more.

Compared with Consciousness I and II, this group contains the highest percentage of women, and is relatively young. They participate in sports and fitness far more than both these groups, but are not satisfied with their current exercise regimen.

A wide majority of Consciousness III types (70%) are likely to claim that they are overweight, and a great many are self-conscious about their physical appearance. They have no particular confidence in their athletic abilities, and by self-assessment, their health ranks somewhat beneath the national norm.

This dominant weight-conscious group is a vast, pent-up reservoir of primed potential converts. A significant number claim to be more interested today in exercise than they were three years ago, and highly receptive to new information about fitness.

Consciousness III fully endorses the concept of physical fitness, expressing many of the same attitudes as the hard-core participant, if not the actual participation behavior. This dominant segment of "Uninitiated Believers" -- comprising 63% of the study sample -- is in essence, the *future of the fitness movement*. Thanks to this group, "Curves for Women" is one of the fastest-growing franchises in American history.

"THE HARD-CORE" -- CONSCIOUSNESS IV

Consciousness IV embraces the ideals of the fitness revolution in both word and deed. Like Consciousness III, they are true believers, but unlike that less motivated group, they are active participants. This hard-core contingent is 57% male, somewhat youthful, distinctively upscale, and the most educated of any segment.

A majority (62%) attain the highest activity level (250+ days per year of sports/fitness participation). 7 out of 10 (71%) watch their diet, while 40% regard their health to be excellent -- compared with 15% for people in general. Not surprisingly, this group is also least likely to smoke cigarettes or to be overweight.

In 2002, this vanguard of the fitness movement accounted for 17% of the U.S. adult population, inching upward from 15% in 1996 and 16% in 1998.

* * *

CHAPTER 7

HEALTH CLUB STRATEGY FOR THE NEW MILLENNIUM: THE PURSUIT OF CONSCIOUSNESS III

In 2002, Health Club members constituted nearly 15% of the adult population, while millions more exercised outdoors, or at home. Including those who worked out at gyms, over 50 million people exercised at least 100 times in a single fitness activity during the year.

Many optimistic Health Club professionals (and marketers of home exercise equipment) naively assume that growth potential for the fitness population must be a simple reciprocal of current penetration; that 85% of the population, for example, are potential health club members. For many reasons, this simplistic view is incorrect:

1. The inactive population includes many who are very old, infirm, disabled or otherwise incapable of physical activity;

2. Many "home" and "outdoors" exercisers are cemented in long-standing fitness habits and are not health club prospects;

3. Millions of potential converts cannot surmount the massive obstacle of inertia…they simply lack self-discipline and require "external" motivation.

On the other hand, despite these limitations and resistances, the "conversion" potential for either health club attendance or home exercise is enormous. To understand why, it is necessary to review the American Sports Data, Inc. segmentation of U.S. Fitness Consciousness, contained in the previous section. As does any topic, Physical Fitness evokes a full range of attitudes and viewpoints -- from inimical detractors to worshipping acolytes; but on this subject, Americans lean heavily toward fitness "enlightenment".

While the prime Consciousness IV segment (Hard-Core exercisers) might or might not be nearing saturation, many of these devotees are set in their ways; some already patronize health clubs, and many are firmly entrenched in home or outdoors exercise. Many are dyed-in-the-wool Runners, Cyclists, Walkers, or veteran exercisers who for years, have been using a Treadmill or Elliptical Trainer at home. This group will not be easily lured to the health club milieu.

A much larger if somewhat less fertile field is the vast expanse of Consciousness III -- the dominant fitness psychographic represented by 128.6 million people across the U.S. These "Uninitiated Believers" have already been converted in spirit; some have begun an exercise routine, and some have even joined a club. They are converts to physical fitness who require only that their receptive attitudes take root in actual fitness behavior.

These data strongly suggest that health club recruitment campaigns focus not on "conversion", but everyday operational incentives (price, convenience, weight loss, per diem rates, dress codes, etc.) that will persuade this already primed group to take that decisive step into the world of fitness. Several million already have made the bold move to "Curves for Women" -- the most successful franchise (of any kind) in American history.

Less active sports/exercise participants (who are not yet health club patrons) account for 40.9 million people within the Consciousness III group. Sedentary individuals in this category -- who have neither a health club affiliation nor an active interest in outdoors or home exercise, but who are also avowed believers -- number 31.9 million prospects (24.8% of Consciousness III).

There are nearly 73 million adult Americans who are favorably disposed toward fitness, but who neither attend a health club nor have any other exercise interest that competes with health club membership. This is the low-hanging fruit.

"Uninitiated Believers" are relatively young, and comprised of a slight majority of women (55%). They are not very active, and tend to worry about three things -- health, bodyweight and the level of stress they endure. These three concerns explain their attraction to fitness and should be the cornerstones of any fitness program catering to Consciousness III.

Of all four psychographic groups, these "Uninitiated Believers" are the least satisfied with their health, have the least flattering perception of their own physicality, and also have the highest rates of diabetes and elevated cholesterol. Consciousness III types feel unhealthy, overweight, lack confidence in their athleticism, and worst of all -- are uncomfortably aware of their physical appearance.

Health monitoring, weight control and stress reduction programs are a must for these "Uninitiated Believers" -- the segment best apprehended by marketing themes that promise less threatening exercise environments. Dress codes, same-gender facilities, mirrorless settings, less demanding exercise forms, user-friendly equipment, fitness pampering and special handholding should be among the basic enticements for these intimidated newcomers.

The phenomenally successful "Curves for Women" format -- already internalized as Express Workouts in many major health club chains -- is a blueprint for the future. And with a 45% male composition, Consciousness III offers huge promise for that gender -- an opportunity already exploited by "Cuts Fitness for Men".

* * *

SPORTS/ACTIVITY PARTICIPATION BY VENUE
TOTAL U.S. POPULATION 18+
(203,876,000)

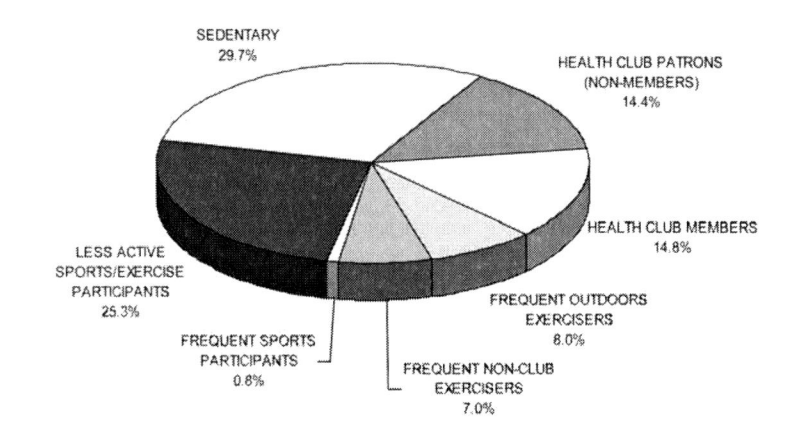

- SEDENTARY 29.7%
- HEALTH CLUB PATRONS (NON-MEMBERS) 14.4%
- HEALTH CLUB MEMBERS 14.8%
- FREQUENT OUTDOORS EXERCISERS 8.0%
- FREQUENT NON-CLUB EXERCISERS 7.0%
- FREQUENT SPORTS PARTICIPANTS 0.8%
- LESS ACTIVE SPORTS/EXERCISE PARTICIPANTS 25.3%

Source: A Comprehensive Study of Consumer Attitudes Toward Physical Fitness and Health Clubs (2002)

"HARD-CORE FITNESS PARTICIPANTS"
FITNESS CONSCIOUSNESS IV
(TOTAL = 34,243,000)

"EXERCISE IS VERY IMPORTANT TO ME, AND I AM A FREQUENT PARTICIPANT IN FITNESS ACTIVITIES"

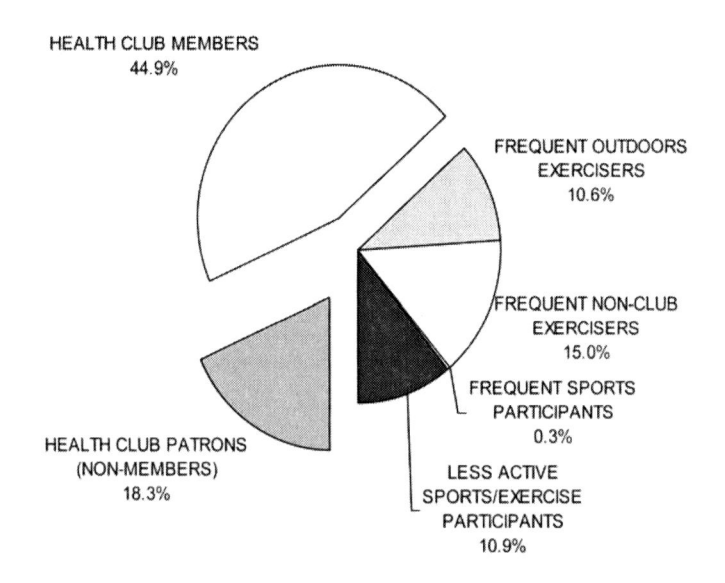

- HEALTH CLUB MEMBERS 44.9%
- FREQUENT OUTDOORS EXERCISERS 10.6%
- FREQUENT NON-CLUB EXERCISERS 15.0%
- FREQUENT SPORTS PARTICIPANTS 0.3%
- LESS ACTIVE SPORTS/EXERCISE PARTICIPANTS 10.9%
- HEALTH CLUB PATRONS (NON-MEMBERS) 18.3%

Source: A Comprehensive Study of Consumer Attitudes Toward Physical Fitness and Health Clubs (2002)

"UNINITIATED BELIEVERS"
FITNESS CONSCIOUSNESS III
(TOTAL = 128,595,000)

"I KNOW EXERCISE IS IMPORTANT, AND I'D LIKE TO PARTICIPATE IN FITNESS ACTIVITIES MORE THAN I DO"

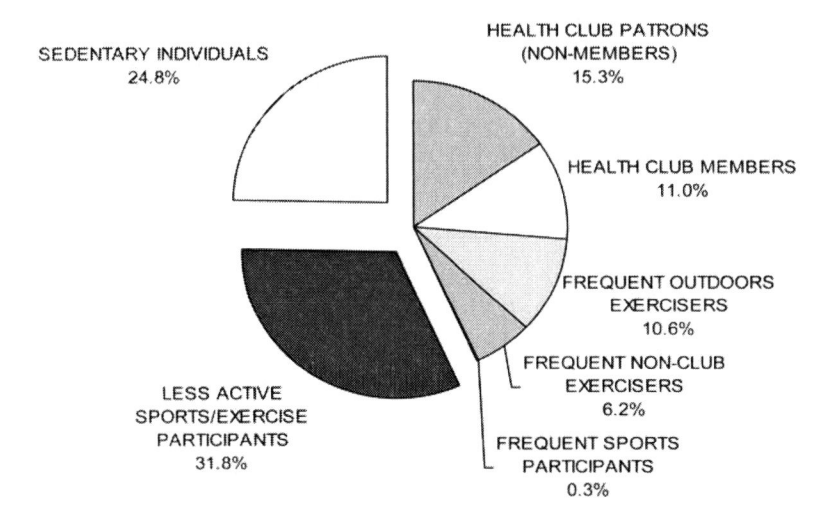

- SEDENTARY INDIVIDUALS — 24.8%
- HEALTH CLUB PATRONS (NON-MEMBERS) — 15.3%
- HEALTH CLUB MEMBERS — 11.0%
- FREQUENT OUTDOORS EXERCISERS — 10.6%
- FREQUENT NON-CLUB EXERCISERS — 6.2%
- FREQUENT SPORTS PARTICIPANTS — 0.3%
- LESS ACTIVE SPORTS/EXERCISE PARTICIPANTS — 31.8%

Source: A Comprehensive Study of Consumer Attitudes Toward Physical Fitness and Health Clubs (2002)

CORRELATES OF FITNESS CONSCIOUSNESS

	I* %	II %	III %	IV %
Female	44	50	55	43
Over 55	24	33	24	31
$75,000+ HH Income	26	18	30	38
College Graduate	16	15	37	49
Sedentary	74	57	25	7
Very Active (250+ sports/fitness days per year)	20	7	15	62
High Stress Level	7	19	28	23
Health is Excellent	26	12	9	38
Overweight	59	59	70	40
Currently on a Diet	3	2	8	5
Smoke Cigarettes	27	36	19	12

* Small sample base

Source: A Comprehensive Study of Consumer Attitudes Toward Physical Fitness and Health Clubs (2002)

SATISFACTION WITH HEALTH & CONDITIONING

	Total Population %	I* %	II %	III %	IV %
Very/Extremely Satisfied					
General State of Health	45	44	47	36	80
Cardio Conditioning	30	31	31	21	66
Physical Strength	33	34	35	24	62
Flexibility	33	28	38	27	53

Level of Fitness Consciousness

* Small sample base

Source: A Comprehensive Study of Consumer Attitudes Toward Physical Fitness and Health Clubs (2002)

MEDICAL CONDITIONS

	Total Population %	Level of Fitness Consciousness			
		I* %	II %	III %	IV %
Asthma/Breathing Disorder	14	18	18	13	6
Arthritis	25	20	30	25	19
Chronic Back Pain	22	25	24	23	13
Diabetes	9	2	7	11	4
Heart Disease	6	2	7	6	9
High Blood Pressure	24	12	25	24	18
High Cholesterol	20	-	14	22	18
Insomnia	14	17	12	15	8

* Small sample base

Source: A Comprehensive Study of Consumer Attitudes Toward Physical Fitness and Health Clubs (2002)

FITNESS ATTITUDES RELATED TO SELF-IMAGE

Level of Fitness Consciousness

Agree	Total Population %	I* %	II %	III %	IV %
I would probably exercise more if I weighed less	32	20	25	38	16
I would prefer to exercise where no one could see me	54	42	58	61	25
I don't have a lot of confidence in my athletic ability	44	41	56	49	17
I would join a health club that catered exclusively to overweight, out-of-shape people like me	32	24	29	37	17
If I had to choose one or the other, I would prefer to lose weight by just dieting, and not doing any exercise	33	59	48	33	14
If I were to join a health club, I would prefer to exercise with members of my own sex, rather than in a "mixed" environment	54	39	62	56	36

* Small sample base

Source: A Comprehensive Study of Consumer Attitudes Toward Physical Fitness and Health Clubs (2002)

CHAPTER 8

PSYCHOLOGICAL STRESS: INVISIBLE PUBLIC HEALTH ENEMY NUMBER ONE

Psychological stress has a decidedly ethereal character. It is invisible, unquantifiable, and practically immeasurable -- pervading our existence like a ghostly fourth dimension. Stress is highly corrosive to our physical and mental health, but because of its intangible nature, we can neither gauge its overall magnitude nor begin to assess its impact on public health, crime, productivity, divorce or countless other social disruptions.

A disturbing 26% of American adult population (53 million people) say that they are experiencing "a lot of stress" in their lives. A little more than half (55%) incur "some stress", while only 16% claim to suffer "no stress at all".

Chronic stress erodes our nervous system, weakens our immune defenses, invites disease and almost certainly shortens the lifespan. But almost none of this has ever been scientifically documented, so for the moment, we must be content with the "softer" proofs of social science.

Powerful correlations between stress and key health indicators consistently point to an unseen gargantuan public health problem -- and imply an immense reward for its antidote. The pharmaceutical companies -- and to a far lesser extent, yoga, biofeedback, and other stress-reduction practitioners -- are already huge beneficiaries.

In our 2002 study, a high level of stress afflicted roughly 1 out of 6 people who reported excellent health (17%), suggesting the existence of "good" stress -- an uncommon, salutary variant. However, the stress factor rises considerably among people who report less than perfect health -- particularly for those who suffer from chronic back pain and insomnia. Not unexpectedly, stress is also related to smoking cigarettes. Of course, it can be argued that poor health in itself is the <u>cause</u> of stress, but the survey question was worded to minimize this possibility.

People who are completely satisfied with various facets of their lives generally suffer less from this pervasive malady than those who are not content. Particularly strong relationships also exist between low stress levels and higher satisfaction with finances, and even more critically -- with the amount of time people have to themselves. Control of one's destiny is also a major correlate of stress.

Those more or less exempt from this latter-day psychological scourge were three times as likely as stress victims (22% - 7%) to be "completely satisfied" with the amount of money they had.

38% of all low-stress respondents were completely satisfied with the amount of time they had for themselves, versus only 11% for the high-stress group.

Two-thirds of people living low-stress lives (67%) felt in control of their destiny, compared with only 31% of those enduring a high degree of stress.

A "blockbuster" correlation was found between reported stress level and one's general psychological state: 48% of all respondents who reported "almost no stress at all in their lives" also claimed complete satisfaction with their "emotional well-being", versus only 11% for the highly-stressed group.

There was only one noticeable deviation from the general pattern: the greatest satisfaction with job/career was reported by people with <u>moderate</u> stress levels -- undoubtedly a rare, productive manifestation of "good" stress.

Powerful correlations were also in evidence between stress level and factors relating to health, fitness and physical self-perception. While 23% of the low-stress group claimed to be completely satisfied with their physical appearance, the number plummeted to 9% among stressed-out individuals.

* * *

"EXPERIENCE A LOT OF STRESS"
(%)

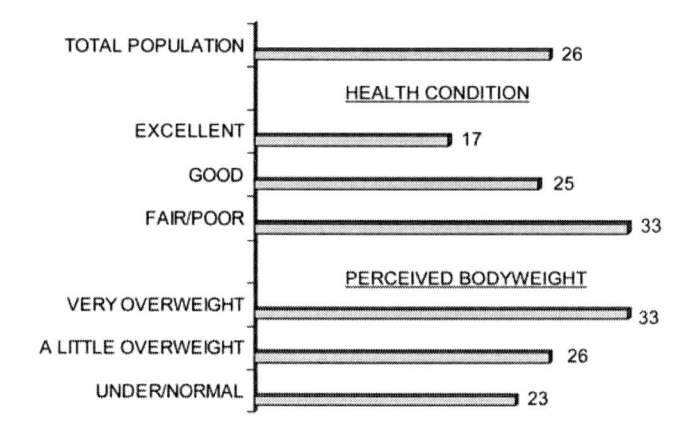

TOTAL POPULATION	26
HEALTH CONDITION	
EXCELLENT	17
GOOD	25
FAIR/POOR	33
PERCEIVED BODYWEIGHT	
VERY OVERWEIGHT	33
A LITTLE OVERWEIGHT	26
UNDER/NORMAL	23

Source: A Comprehensive Study of Consumer Attitudes Toward Physical Fitness and Health Clubs (2002).

STRESS LEVEL BY HEALTH CONDITION

STRESS LEVEL

Suffer From:	Total %	High %	Moderate %	Low %
Arthritis	25	25	25	28
Chronic Back Pain	22	30	18	21
Hypertension	24	24	22	28
High Cholesterol	20	24	18	21
Asthma/Breathing Disorder	14	18	12	14
Insomnia	14	22	12	9
Heart Disease	6	4	7	8
Diabetes	9	8	10	6
Smoke Cigarettes	21	30	19	15

Source: A Comprehensive Study of Consumer Attitudes Toward Physical Fitness and Health Clubs (2002).

SATISFACTION WITH LIFESTYLE
BY LEVEL OF PSYCHOLOGICAL STRESS

	Total Population %	High Stress %	Moderate Stress %	Low Stress %
Completely Satisfied With…:				
The way my job or career is going	18	11	22	16
The amount of time I have to myself	20	11	19	38
My friendships	37	28	38	49
The amount of money I have	13	7	13	22
My relationship with my spouse or significant other	44	37	45	51
My relationship with my family	49	38	50	64
Keeping stress at a reasonable level	17	7	16	37
My emotional well-being	26	11	26	48
I Have Control Over My Destiny (8-10 rating ~ on 1-10 scale)	44	31	42	67

Source: A Comprehensive Study of Consumer Attitudes Toward Physical Fitness and Health Clubs (2002).

COMPLETE SATISFACTION WITH ASPECTS OF LIFE
BY LEVEL OF PSYCHOLOGICAL STRESS

Completely Satisfied With…:	Total Population %	High Stress %	Moderate Stress %	Low Stress %
My physical health	15	8	16	23
My physical appearance	13	9	12	23
My physical fitness	9	5	10	9
The amount and quality of exercise I get	11	7	11	15
Maintaining a healthful diet	14	10	12	22
My weight	15	9	15	20

Source: A Comprehensive Study of Consumer Attitudes Toward Physical Fitness and Health Clubs (2002).

CHAPTER 9

KINDER, GENTLER FITNESS TRENDS CONTINUE TO DISPLACE TRADITIONAL EXERCISE FORMS

FOR IMMEDIATE RELEASE   April 15, 2003

* * *

Pilates, Elliptical Trainers, Recumbent Bikes and Yoga are Fastest-Growing Activities

HARTSDALE, N.Y. -- To accommodate legions of newly-arrived converts who are older, female, or both, less strenuous exercise forms and user-friendly equipment are fanning out over the landscape of physical fitness -- in some cases sweeping aside more vigorous pursuits originally aimed at the "traditional" participant. Since 1998, the top growth activities have been Pilates Training, Elliptical Motion Trainers, Recumbent Cycling and Yoga -- activities with generally older and female constituencies. These were among the findings of the 16th annual Superstudy® of Sports Participation, conducted in January 2003 among 15,063 people nationwide, by American Sports Data, Inc. (ASD).

Pilates, a hybrid resistance/balance/stretching exercise which lay dormant for the better part of a century, has resurfaced to claim 4.7 million participants nationwide -- a 92% increase over the 2001 measurement of 2.4 million. In 2002, the newly-minted activity continues to be dominated by women, who account for 90% of all participants; 67% of all Pilates exercisers were first-year participants. Many Pilates and Yoga practitioners will rail violently against the notion -- implied or otherwise -- that these are "easy" activities.

The Elliptical Motion Trainer -- described as a cross between a Nordic Ski Machine and Stair Climber -- is a particularly friendly exercise to those with knee problems. By 2002, it had attracted 10.7 million participants, a surge of 177% over the 1998 benchmark of 3.9 million. Unlike certain short-lived predecessors (i.e. Nordic Skiers, Aerobic Riders) which were sustained by infomercials, Elliptical Trainers have passed the litmus test of Health Club acceptance -- the imprimatur which guarantees the future of fitness equipment.

According to other ASD research, 26% of the U.S. population claims to be experiencing "a lot of stress" in their lives. It is therefore no surprise that the compound measurement of Yoga/Tai Chi reflects an increase of 95% from 1998 - 2002. Yoga -- emblematic of the new genre of mind-body relaxation techniques which defy traditional categorization as "fitness" activities -- claimed 11.1 million adherents in 2002, 83% of whom were female.

Overshadowed by a far more glamorous younger sibling, Recumbent Cycling has gone virtually unnoticed. Yet, this robust growth activity has exploded to 10.2 million participants -- an increase of 51% from 1998. By contrast, the far more publicized activity of Spinning has declined by 10% during this period, registering only 6.1 million participants in 2002.

Strength-training -- once the exclusive male preserve of muscle-bound jocks -- has not only earned universal acceptance, but made its largest gains among women and older fitness enthusiasts. Women now constitute 47% of all people who train with free weights, and command an identical percentage of Weight/Resistance Machine-users. Both Free Weights and Weight Machines are strong growth categories.

Treadmill exercise epitomizes "kinder/gentler" fitness. From its fledgling measurement of 4.4 million in 1987, a record of 43.4 million participants in 2002 marks 15 years of uninterrupted growth – a quantum leap of 888%, including a still-vibrant 17% growth rate since 1998. Treadmill usage is the most popular cardiovascular exercise in the U.S.; 59% of its practitioners are female, 38% over the age of 45.

Aerobics and Cardio Kickboxing represent the more "traditional" fitness activities that have lost ground in recent years… arguably victims of newer, less taxing forms of exercise. From its initial measurement of 7.6 million in 1999, Kickboxing has plummeted 22% to 5.9 million in 2002. All variations of Aerobic Dancing continue their downward spiral, dipping to a low of 16 million participants; the original High-Impact version has plunged to 5.4 million dancers in 2002, down 61% from the 1987 baseline measurement of 14 million.

From 1998 - 2002, major losses have been sustained in three other categories: Stair-Climbers (-23%); Nordic Ski Machines (-26%); Aerobic Riders (-38%).

While these newer, less taxing fitness forms have an "older" skew than traditional "hardbody" pursuits -- Pilates, Yoga, and Treadmill Exercise have the demographic diversity to absorb youthful defectors from Cardio Kickboxing, Step-Aerobics and other more rigorous but declining activities. For the year 2000, Pilates exercisers registered an average age of 43.6; by 2002 the mean had declined to 35.1 years. Similarly, the age of a Yoga practitioner had declined from 41.5 in 1998 to 37.1 in 2002.

But regardless of changing exercise preferences, the fitness industry knows it can rely on a perennial ally: the growing consensus among fitness enthusiasts -- tacit or otherwise -- is that they need outside motivation, discipline, know-how, and maybe even a little handholding. In 2002, Health Club membership across the U.S. reached a record-high 36,289,000 -- an increase of 23% over 1998, and a jump of 109% from its 1987 benchmark. 6 million people paid for the services of a Personal Trainer in 2002, up a full 50% from 1998.

The Superstudy® of Sports Participation was conducted in January 2003 and based on a nationally representative sample of 15,063 people over the age of 6 who were among 25,000 respondents targeted in a sample drawn from the consumer mail panel of NFO Research, Inc. 103 sports and activities were measured along over 20 demographic, attitudinal and behavioral dimensions. Data were also collected on health club membership and other subjects pertinent to physical fitness. This annual tracking study has been conducted by ASD every year since 1987, and sponsored by the Sporting Goods Manufacturers Association of North Palm Beach, Florida. For more information, log onto www.americansportsdata.com.

* * *

SELECTED FITNESS ACTIVITIES

Participated at least once (000) 1998-2002

	1998	1999	2000	2001	2002	1-Year Change 2001-2002	4-Year Change 1998-2002
Pilates Training	n.a.	n.a.	1,739	2,437	4,671	+92%	+169%[1]
Elliptical Motion Trainers	3,863	5,081	6,176	8,255	10,695	+30%	+177%
Yoga/Tai Chi	5,708	6,404	7,400	9,741	11,106	+14%	+95%
Stationary Cycling (Recumbent)	6,773	9,771	8,947	8,654	10,217	+18%	+51%
Weight/Resistance Machines	22,519	22,961	25,182	25,942	27,848	+7%	+24%
Dumbbells	23,414	24,754	25,241	26,773	28,933	+8%	+24%
Hand Weights	23,325	25,862	27,086	27,078	28,453	+5%[†]	+22%
Home Gym Exercise	7,577	7,918	8,103	8,497	8,924	+5%[†]	+18%
Barbells	21,263	21,717	21,972	23,030	24,812	+8%	+17%
Treadmill Exercise	37,073	37,463	40,816	41,638	43,431	+4%	+17%
Stretching	35,114	35,278	36,408	38,120	38,367	+1%[†]	+9%
Ab Machine/Device	16,534	17,109	18,119	18,692	17,370	-7%[†]	+5%

[†] Statistically insignificant at the 95% Confidence Level

SOURCE: AMERICAN SPORTS DATA, INC.

SELECTED FITNESS ACTIVITIES (Continued)

Participated at least once (000) 1998-2002

	1998	1999	2000	2001	2002	1-Year Change 2001-2002	4-Year Change 1998-2002
Aquatic Exercise	6,685	5,557	6,367	7,103	6,995	- 2%[†]	+ 5%[†]
Fitness Walking	36,395	35,976	36,207	36,445	37,981	+ 4%[†]	+ 4%[†]
Running/Jogging	34,962	34,047	33,680	34,857	35,866	+ 3%[†]	+ 3%[†]
Swimming (Laps/Fitness)	15,258	14,194	14,060	15,300	14,542	- 5%[†]	- 5%[†]
Stationary Cycling (Spinning)	6,776	6,945	5,431	6,418	6,135	- 4%[†]	- 10%[†]
Stationary Cycling (Upright Bike)	20,744	18,311	17,894	17,483	17,403	- 1%[†]	- 16%
Fitness Biking (Outdoors)	13,556	12,307	11,435	10,761	11,153	+ 4%[†]	- 18%
Cardio Kickboxing	n.a.	7,607	7,163	6,665	5,940	-11%[†]	-22%[2]
Stair Climbers	18,609	16,288	15,828	15,117	14,251	- 6%[†]	- 23%
Aerobics (Net)	21,017	19,129	17,326	16,948	16,046	- 5%[†]	- 24%
X-C Ski Machines	6,870	5,921	5,444	4,924	5,074	+ 3%[†]	- 26%
Aerobic Riders	5,868	4,165	3,817	3,918	3,654	- 7%[†]	- 38%

[1] 2-year Change
[2] 3-year Change

SOURCE: AMERICAN SPORTS DATA, INC.

CHAPTER 10

THE FUTURE OF FITNESS

The contemporary Fitness Movement carries the DNA of the 1960's counterculture, which -- among many other "radical" values -- gave rise to a new focus on psychological and physical self-improvement. Physical self-enhancement branched off on its own, evolving into one of the most dramatic cultural changes of the 20th century -- the Fitness Revolution. This remarkable history begins with the running boom of the 1970's, and in the racquet-dominated "health clubs" of the same decade; it then proceeds to the aerobics boomlet of the early 1980's, and a few years later, ushers in a third generation of low-impact activities, such as Fitness Walking, Soft Aerobics and Treadmill exercise. Low-impact is the real revolution, because it makes fitness available to <u>everyone</u>.

In the 1990's, physical fitness began to redefine itself -- both demographically and topically. The new exploding genre of easier, potentially less strenuous, or otherwise user-friendly equipment included Steppers, Recumbent Bikes, light Hand-Weights, and -- toward the end of the decade -- Elliptical Trainers. More than 20% of all Health Club members were now over 55 years of age.

By the turn of the Millennium, the megatrend of physical fitness had lost its 1970's innocence. Many of the spartan gyms of that era were replaced by lavish fitness palaces; and coming full circle, Weight Training (the proto-activity of the original health club) had returned to rival CV exercise as a dominant fitness form. But the most important contemporary subtrend is probably the new genre of kinder and gentler fitness: stretching, flexibility, balance and relaxation techniques. By integrating the mental and physical, some of these new mind-body incarnations defy traditional categorization as "fitness" activities.

In 2003, most Americans are persuaded that physical activity is essential to good health, and over 50 million adults are frequent exercisers, participating over 100 times a year in at least one fitness activity. From a baseline of near-zero in 1950, a logarithmic curve makes the near-vertical ascent to a fitness utopia of 2050: daily workouts are the norm for every able-bodied American; and those who desist are social outcasts. Long after universal healthcare is established, an unforeseen blend of futuristic values and incentivized physical fitness will usher in an era of near-universal physical fitness participation. Nearly everyone will exercise.

But there is a competing scenario in which people <u>never</u> exercise. In this alternative future, technology -- for centuries the natural enemy of physical activity -- is finally triumphant, inventing a "magic pill" which supplies all nutriment, prevents weight gain, and otherwise ensures perfect health.

Naturally, drugs cannot replace the essence of physical activity, and reality will be far more complicated than science fiction. While a sizeable element of the U.S. population currently favors a magical weight loss drug, the threat of such a Viagra-like bombshell appears -- at least momentarily -- to be subsiding. In 1996, 46% of the population endorsed such a hypothetical panacea; by 2002, support had eroded to 38%.

But neither is there evidence (as of this writing) that Americans are becoming more physical. In 2002 there were 50.9 million frequent exercisers -- nearly identical to the 51.5 million reported in 1990. On a per capita basis the percentage of frequent fitness participants in the U.S. has declined from 23.2% to 19.8%. Far worse (as the media informs us daily), American eating habits are out of control -- and the country is on the brink of an obesity epidemic. Ironically, people have finally recognized their need for structure, information, stimulation and external discipline; and in the midst of a stalled fitness movement -- Health Clubs and Personal Trainers -- the two venues that address these needs, are flourishing.

All this sounds (and is) confusing, but the immediate future of fitness is relatively straightforward. While the vast majority of Americans are fitness-conscious, behavior continues to lag enlightened attitudes -- a finding which replicates the surveys of 1996 and 1998. 80% of all Americans are sold on the idea of fitness, but only 17% describe themselves as Hard-Core Participants -- dubbed "Consciousness IV" in the study.

The majority of Americans (63%) recognize the importance of being fit, but don't get enough exercise. This "Consciousness III" segment, tagged "Uninitiated Believers", represents the future of both the Health Club industry and exercise equipment business. The new fitness prospect is overweight, unathletic, self-conscious, intimidated, and not surprisingly…requires easier exercise, user-friendly equipment and lots of handholding! The spoils will go to the Health Club chains and/or Fitness equipment marketers that satisfy these criteria.

Consciousness II types are "Indifferent", while Consciousness I (only 2% of the population) depicts the near-extinct species of "Non-Believers". Neither group is important to Fitness marketing.

The future of Fitness is festooned with delightful inventions: advanced interactive virtual reality, futuristic physiological monitoring (sunglasses that decipher retinal patterns, for example), remote heart rate sensors, extremely sophisticated electronic logs and training schedules combined with remote healthcare management, very "smart" wireless technology that links home fitness and personal entertainment preferences with any health club in the world, and so on. But only one prediction can be made with certainty: innovation -- science fiction-like or otherwise -- must increase human perspiration. Otherwise, it is for naught.

* * *

CHAPTER 11

FITNESS *AND* FATNESS BOOM?

THE NEW AMERICAN PARADOX:
EXERCISE AND THE BALLOONING OF A NATION

The New Human Condition

For tens of thousands of years, starvation was the natural human condition. Chiseled by scarcity and hunger, the human body was very likely an unpleasing silhouette of gauntness, desiccation and distention. But in prehistoric times, people had no choices.

Today we have many choices, and superabundance in the Third Millennium has abolished the unsightly pre-historic figure -- but only to evolve an equally displeasing profile of flesh, girth and rotundity. To be sure, the new American form does not portend the brief life expectancy of our ancestors; but the evidence is mounting that obesity will shorten our lives and undercut the quality of much longer life spans promised by souped-up medical science of the 21st century. And most remarkably, our new national figure has been cut within the last twenty years -- well after the "me-decade" of the 1970's and the paradigm shift we call the fitness boom.

With overwhelming statistical evidence, the Surgeon General has proclaimed an obesity epidemic in the United States. A national survey conducted in 2002 by American Sports Data, Inc. revealed that 61% of all adults in the U.S. felt that they were overweight, 19% admitting that they were "considerably" overweight. In 2001, the Centers for Disease Control (CDC) -- using a more rigorous self-report measure of "Body Mass Index" (a ratio of bodyweight to height) in the Behavioral Risk Factor Surveillance System (BRFSS) -- determined that by virtue of a 30.0+ BMI, 21% of the population is obese. This is in stark contrast to 1991, when only 12% of the population was so categorized. In the even more objective National Health and Nutrition Examination Survey (where people's height and weight are actually measured), obesity levels soar upward of 30%. 5% of all people are <u>extremely</u> obese, as are 15% of all Black women.

To the extent that children represent our future, the findings are even more dismal. According to the CDC, the percentage of overweight children 6-11 has nearly <u>doubled</u> since the early 1980's, while the percentage of overweight adolescents has almost <u>tripled</u>.

The Surgeon General has further declared obesity responsible for 300,000 deaths every year -- a toll surpassed only by tobacco, to which 400,000 deaths are attributed. If this budding epidemiological nightmare is not a sufficient wake-up call, we have an even more provocative statistic: the most commonly purchased woman's dress size in America is 14. In 1985, it was a size 8!

Goliath Casket is a specialty manufacturer of oversize coffins. Since the company's inception in the late 1980's, sales of its triple-wide models have increased exponentially.

The airline industry has been warned to factor in the increasing

American bodyweight in the calculation of maximum loads. Some restaurants are adding inches to chairs…Enough said.

Obesity and the Anti-Smoking Campaign: Déjà Vu All Over Again
Begun in earnest with the original 1964 Surgeon General's Report on smoking, the obesity scourge of 2003 has an historic parallel -- the war on tobacco. This famous clarion call decreed smoking hazardous to one's health, and -- in a judgment reserved for future medical historians -- ranks as a supreme landmark in the history of public health. The analogy is irresistible; if smoking cessation has saved millions of lives, the conquest of obesity may garner equal glory in the pantheon of public health. Surgeon General Satcher's 2001 report on obesity went practically unnoticed; but neither was the initial volley of the 1964 report on smoking heard round the world. It took several years to rouse public opinion and muster the anti-smoking campaigns that ultimately raised American consciousness.

The similarities between smoking and the overweight condition end here. Both remedies require discipline, but smoking cessation is a simple binary, on-off proposition. Weight loss is more complicated; we can't simply "stop eating".

The obesity epidemic is well-documented, but not fully documented. Its origins remain complex. We know that excess food intake minus inadequately compensating physical activity equals increasing average bodyweight; but beyond this simple physical calculus, no one has offered a cogent, comprehensive explanation for the Ballooning of America. Just as America's plummeting crime rate remains the greatest unsolved sociological mystery of the late 20th century, the rise of the obesity epidemic in America emerges as a great riddle of the early 21st.

Obesity and the Falling Crime Rate: The Search for "Superfactors"
From 1994 - 2002, violent crime victimization rates in the U.S. plunged by 55%, the massive decline cutting a nearly equal swath across urban, suburban and rural areas.

Is there a mayor or police chief in the country who has not taken credit for the drop in crime -- so eerily uniform throughout the land? A new resolve to fight crime, beefed-up law enforcement budgets and other efforts certainly contributed to the mysteriously waning crime rate; but so did other factors, such as an improved economy, favorable demographic trends, a rising prison population (fewer criminals on the streets) and a disappearing crack epidemic. And now Steven Levitt, a pragmatic, untraditional young economist at the University of Chicago drops an analytical bombshell -- Roe v. Wade. Legalized abortion, says this refreshingly bold thinker, was an unmistakable antecedent of a falling crime rate 15-20 years hence. His thesis is stunning, macabre and elegant: the millions of unborn babies in the wake of Roe v. Wade were precisely the unwanted children and high-risk demographics, that -- had they come to term -- would have committed the crimes! Levitt's theory has absorbed the full gamut of abuse and acclaim: simplistic, wrong-headed and repugnant; also ingenious, brilliant and seminal. The superfactor underlying the falling crime rate may be crack, abortion or just simple economics…Crime may be <u>inversely related to the rising tide that lifts all boats</u>: the constantly improved condition of Americans -- contrarian reports notwithstanding.

Compared with crime, the phenomenon of obesity at first seems an easy subject to dissect and quantify, but ultimately proves to be a more complex subject for analysis. The superfactor that explains obesity may be overeating -- but neither is that a certainty.

Root Causes of Overweight and Obesity: Peripheral Suspects

Were Levitt to train his socioeconomic lens on the obesity question, he would magnify a daunting problem -- one more complex and much less conducive to the type of dominant-factor, blockbuster solution that according to his divination, now explains at least 50 percent of the drop in crime. He could easily identify the familiar lineup of suspects, but in 2003, forensic social analysis cannot yet produce hard evidence:

- <u>Genetics</u>…Fat people beget fat children…and unless the environment is to blame -- there isn't a thing anyone can do about it. But changes in DNA structure caused by mutation take a lot longer than 20 years; so we need to look elsewhere for the root causes of a recent obesity epidemic.

- <u>Population Trends</u>…If certain overweight segments of the population (i.e. Hispanics, low-income groups, senior citizens) are growing faster than the general population, we have some easily identifiable correlates of obesity, but still no root causes.

- <u>Harried Lifestyles</u>…Working Moms, Single Dads and a generally time-starved populace have fueled the take-in, eat-out and particularly, the fast-food industries. With half of all food budgets spent outside the home, there is no question that the obsolescence of the traditional dinner table has taken a toll on health and bodyweight. But how much?

- <u>High-Carbohydrate Diets</u>…A shibboleth of the fitness boom of the 70's and 80's was a low-fat, high-carbohydrate diet -- not an easy way to lose weight, we now realize. With the star of the late Dr. Atkins now very high in the firmament, eating habits are already changing. Not all agree, but the new trendiness toward high-protein diets may be one of the few bright spots on the horizon.

- <u>A Less Demanding Workplace?</u>…While technology has always been the natural enemy of physical activity, this favorite adage rings most true from the Industrial Revolution to about the 1950's and 1960's. Since that time, technology has continued to eradicate manual labor, shifting millions of jobs to a physically undemanding service sector. But paradoxically, the surviving legions of a once-trim blue-collar army (donut-munching policemen and beer-quaffing ironworkers) are less fit than their sedentary upscale counterparts! White-collar jobs may be proliferating, may require a lower caloric expenditure, but in the present social context, desk workers -- though theoretically at risk -- are not inordinate casualties.

- <u>Smoking Cessation</u>…Weight gain is an immutable law of smoking cessation: quit smoking, add avoirdupois. According to the CDC, in 2001 ex-smokers registered an obesity rate of 23.9% versus only 17.8% for current smokers. Since 1979, smoking has declined from 33% of the adult population to 22% in 2002, so we have apprehended another minor (but clearly guilty) offender.

Poetically, the greatest triumph in the history of public health (the anti-smoking campaign), becomes a minor impediment to a second monumental challenge 40 years later! Indeed, this offender is by far the most noble of obesity villains.

Fitness and Fatness Boom

- <u>TV: The All-Purpose Whipping Boy</u>...In that people who watch a great deal of television are physically "heavier" than those who spend fewer hours so engaged, TV viewing is said to be "related" to obesity. But these two factors are also intercorrelated with other surrogate variables such as income, fitness behavior and food consumption -- any one of which pre-empts the "causal" relationship thought to exist between TV watching and being overweight. In other words, it is true that fat people spend more time in front of the tube than leaner ones; but it is equally true that less affluent households log more TV time, and that less affluent households have higher obesity rates than their upscale counterparts. It can therefore be argued that people are transfixed to the TV screen simply because they have less income and education -- and <u>not</u> because they also happen to weigh more than less rabid TV viewers. Socioeconomic status may be the key driver of <u>both</u> TV-watching <u>and</u> obesity, but remarkably, this sloppy muddle of correlation and causality has never been challenged.

Television is also accused of breeding physical inactivity and encouraging that most insidious form of overeating -- snacking. Yet overall trends in TV viewership are absolutely uncorrelated with recent gains in American girth. In 1988, according to Nielsen Media Research, adult males watched television an average of 3 hours and 59 minutes per day; for women, the mean was 4:41. By 2001, the numbers were 4:19 and 4:51: respective increases of 8% and 4% -- certainly not enough to implicate TV in the adult obesity crisis.

For children, TV time has actually declined during this period. From 1988 - 2001 teenage viewing dropped from 3:18 per day to 3:04, while younger children reflected a similar fall-off -- from 3:22 to 3:12. Naturally, all of this slack (and probably more) has been absorbed by the internet, CD's, video games and email -- activities which may be less amenable to snacking.

In any case, for no age group is there even a remote causal connection between TV viewing and obesity. Social class -- not necessarily TV -- is the miscreant. We can't blame television any more than the automobile -- they've both been around too long!

- <u>Social Class</u>…The relationship between social rank and body type is not a recent discovery. As early as 1983, in a snippy, but erudite sociological treatise/pop culture funbook titled "Class", Paul Fussell observed that both humans and canines who inhabit the upper crust of society are far leaner than those in the lower strata.

Less amusingly, recent indicators point to a widening of this paradoxical gap between have's and have nots…For Black and Hispanic Inner-City populations, a growing reliance on junk food, the absence of nutritional counseling and a dearth of preventive medical care add up to a greater-than-average risk for both obesity and general health problems.

A Strong Contender: The Unraveling of American Discipline?
America started gaining weight in the early 1980's, and has been adding poundage ever since. Our first instinct -- and it may turn out to be the correct one -- is to blame our rising per capita food intake; as a nation, we're just eating more and more. But then there's another guilty-looking suspect -- physical inactivity. We could simply correlate physical fitness participation with weight gain over the past 20 years, and quickly trap the culprit…<u>if</u> we had reliable and consistent survey data reaching back to 1980.

Quite remarkably, even after such major initiatives as the 1996 Report of the Surgeon General on Physical Activity and Health,

Fitness and Fatness Boom

Healthy People 2000, and Healthy People 2010, fitness research remains a very low governmental priority. The well-known "national health" studies conducted by the Federal Government touch upon fitness behavior, but these efforts are sporadic -- with inconsistent methodologies that all but negate their tracking value. Indeed, this monumental public health concern is not deemed worthy of dedicated, on-going tracking research that would monitor the nation's progress (or lack thereof) in this vital area of preventive healthcare. For example, the best federal tracking estimate of physical activity (BRFSS) begins in 1990, does not include children, and asks respondents <u>only about the two physical activities</u> they engage in most often.

This informational void has been partially filled by American Sports Data, Inc. which noted that from 1987 - 1990, the fitness boom was still climbing -- presumably along an upward trajectory launched ten years earlier. But from 1980 - 1990, according to the CDC, <u>Americans gained weight -- *concurrent* with rising levels of fitness behavior</u>.

According to annual tracking surveys initiated in 1987 by American Sports Data, Inc., the fitness revolution reached its apogee in 1990. Since that time, the number of frequent fitness participants in the U.S. has fallen imperceptibly from 51 million in 1990, to 50.9 million in 2002. But factoring out population growth, there has been a per capita decline of 15% in frequent fitness participation (100+ days per year in any one activity). Among children 12-17, the plunge is 41% -- hard evidence of a monumental neglect that mirrors the dilapidated state of physical education in U.S. public schools.

A more comprehensive approach factoring in all recreational sports as well as fitness activities reveals only a minor fall in aggregate per capita participation days -- from 159 in 1990, to 153 in 2002 -- a drop of 4%. But for children aged 6-17, the decline is much sharper -- a plunge of 11% in just 4 years. For older Americans (55+), per capita participation has increased 12% from 1998 - 2002, raising the not so tongue-in-cheek suggestion that grandparents may soon be fitter than grandchildren.

Obviously, this methodology is based on only the total number of days of reported activity, and does not attempt to measure how long or hard people exercise -- two factors essential to the quantification of total energy expenditure. Nor does ASD research account for the calories people burn outside of structured sports/fitness behavior. Still, even in a state of perfect quantification, the existing hypothesis would probably not be threatened: for the entire population, per capita sports/fitness activity (and therefore caloric expenditure) has declined somewhat since 1990 -- but not nearly enough to account for the fattening of America. And it is doubtful that the casual, informal, unstructured physical activity required from work, daily chores or any other aspect of everyday living would compensate for the drop in sports/fitness behavior.   If anything, the vanishing energy requirement of mundane, routine behavior is contributing to the sedentary lifestyle; but according to the scant, fragmentary evidence available from CDC studies, overall inactivity trends cannot begin to explain the magnitude of our obesity problem.

While these data do suggest a flagging of the national spirit, our collective fitness-consciousness is highly evolved and surprisingly strong. In three separate tracking studies since 1996, ASD has documented that while only 20% of the population are frequent exercisers, many more (around 80% of all adults) are persuaded of the virtues of fitness, and most think they should exercise more. To bolster a weakening resolve, millions of Americans -- in the face of an overall lackluster fitness movement -- are flocking to Health Clubs and Personal Trainers. Health Club membership in the U.S. now stands at 36.3 million, dwarfing the 1987 count of 17.4 million by 109%. In 2002, 5.4 million Americans paid for the services of a personal trainer -- up 30% since 1999.

Physical fitness activity, as it relates to bodyweight, is a complex issue. For the 1990's, we have a slight erosion of sports/fitness behavior, rising obesity levels, but at the same time -- a major plea for help, evidenced by skyrocketing health club and personal trainer usage. Americans are very fitness-conscious, but are constantly struggling to overcome a perennial lack of discipline. Fitness behavior simply lags enlightened attitudes.

The coin of discipline has a flipside -- food consumption. Tracking data are unavailable, but according to American Sports Data, Inc., in 2002, 7 out of 10 adults (72%) attempted either to lose at least five pounds or maintain their present weight. Only 7% went on a formal diet, while 49% claimed to "watch what they ate" as a weight control strategy. While a fairly large percentage reported short-term success, only 30% of those who attempted to lose weight through dieting or physical activity were able to keep off the excess poundage.

The Prime Candidate: Overconsumption

In the war on obesity, American discipline is hopelessly overmatched by two formidable adversaries: superabundance and mega marketing.

Greg Critser, author of "Fat Land", has popularized the idea of a gigantic corn surplus as the lowest common denominator (if not dominant superfactor) behind the current obesity epidemic.

Now, as in Revolutionary times, a massive surfeit of corn is responsible for a great societal ill. Two hundred years ago -- to the great moral detriment of an impressionable young nation -- the same cornucopia was distilled into a huge overabundance of cheap corn whiskey.

Today, the nearly infinite largess of corn is distilled into limitless quantities of high-fructose corn syrup, resulting in much larger bottles of Coke and Pepsi at still-affordable prices. Cheap corn -- converted to both animal feed and direct food ingredients -- is a cornerstone of profitability for various other industries: processed foods, chicken, beef and fast-food, to name a few.

Rather than grace the American people with lower prices, courtesy of this dirt-cheap commodity, Big Food has callously rebuffed a rare public service opportunity in favor of the bottom line. Instead of cutting prices, food companies opt to increase profits by making more food available.

Agribusiness, according to Dr. Marion Nestle, Professor and Chair of the Department of Nutrition and Food Studies at New

Fitness _and_ Fatness Boom

York University, now produces 3,800 calories of food a day for every American, 500 calories more than 30 years ago -- but at much lower per-calorie costs. Fast food restaurants are multiple blights on every zip code in the U.S., while food conglomerates are force-feeding a none-too-reluctant population calorie-packed meals with larger portion sizes. The Public Health Service -- aided and abetted by the food lobby -- has, in the past, deliberately suppressed reports issuing "unfavorable" guidelines; unfavorable that is, in the recommendation of lower food consumption or selected food products. U.S. food and beverage giants have transformed school cafeterias into fattening pens, breeding a gargantuan health problem which now, is merely an epidemic; but when our children reach maturity, it may evolve another order of magnitude -- to public health disaster!

But repentance may be at hand. McDonald's, Kraft, and Coca-Cola -- in the early stages of social awareness -- are planning to mend their ways. Presumably, other industry behemoths are also on the fast-track to redemption, which is of course, is far more important than whether or not a Steven Levitt ever officially indicts the arch-villain of this impending public health calamity.

* * *

CHAPTER 12

NATIONWIDE HEALTH CONCERNS MAY BE PUMPING U.S. FITNESS BEHAVIOR

FOR IMMEDIATE RELEASE   April 20, 2004

* * *

Over 39 million Americans now belong to Health Clubs, and many more are Frequent Fitness Participants, New Study finds

* * *

Kinder/Gentler Exercise in an Unintimidating Venue is the key for many -- but will it tame the National Waistline?

HARTSDALE, N.Y. -- Americans have been fitness-conscious for some time...but now there is evidence that a growing national awareness is finally inspiring many to action. Galvanized by widespread media coverage of the obesity epidemic, Big Foods' promise of reduced portion sizes and less fat content, new fitness-based premium incentives by HMO's -- and most fascinatingly, legislative murmurs about a new social contract between government and taxpaying fitness participants -- millions of tentative Americans could finally be making that long-delayed leap from enlightenment to actual fitness behavior.

A consistent finding of studies conducted by American Sports Data, Inc. (ASD) in 1996, 1998 and 2002 is that over 80% of the adult population pays homage to the ideal of physical fitness, while only one in five gets enough exercise, a fraction that -- due to nullifying gains and losses in a wide range of fitness activities (and despite continually rising health club memberships) -- has remained constant over the years. But there is evidence that this is changing.

According to the seventeenth annual SUPERSTUDY® of Sports participation, 54.9 million people who engaged in a single fitness activity on at least 100 occasions. While this measurement includes the new genre of "Mind-Body" exercise (and is therefore not comparable with prior estimates), "same-sport" comparisons indicate an overall increase in frequent exercise. In addition, the study projected 39.4 million health club members -- an increase of 8.6% over the previous year. While part of this increase is attributable to random statistical variation, substantial membership growth is supported by independent data. A nationwide compilation of Yellow Pages listings by InfoUSA enumerates 23,497 clubs as of January 1, 2004 -- an increase of 16% over the prior year tally of 20,207. According to ASD president Harvey Lauer, "70% of all Yellow Pages listings are bona fide Commercial Health Clubs -- not YMCA's, Gymnastics studios or Personal Trainers -- and this increment of over 3,000 new facilities by itself accounts for a good portion of several million additional club members. A modest growth rate of even 4% among pre-existing chains could account for the remainder."

As flagship of the Mind-Body fitness movement, Pilates

Training is far and away the "hottest" growth trend, according to the new ASD report. With 9.5 million participants in 2003, this hybrid stretching/resistance activity has grown by 103% in just the past year, and by 445% from its initial measurement of 1.7 million in 1998. 89% of Pilates practitioners are female.

Elliptical Motion Trainers continue their upward trajectory, garnering 13.4 million participants in 2003, up 25% for the year, and 247% since 1998. While users of these machines are not particularly old (average age 36.5), this equipment, among other virtues, is "knee-friendly" -- a clear qualification for the Kinder/Gentler category. Elliptical Trainers are also the only conceivable long-term threat to Treadmill Exercise.

With an average age of 43.5 and 48.3 for frequent participants (100+ days), Recumbent Cycling is the second "eldest" exercise activity -- trailing only Fitness Walking in participant longevity. Since 1998, this "back-friendly" variation on the Kinder/Gentler theme has increased by 58%, to 10.7 million participants.

The compound measurement of Yoga/Tai Chi claimed 13.4 million adherents in 2003, a growth rate of 20% for the current year, and 134% since 1998. Like Pilates, Yoga has a large female following: 78%.

Treadmill Exercise, the largest single physical fitness activity and once a Roman candle -- has slowed to lumbering, but inexorable single-digit growth. With 45.6 million participants in 2003 -- a Vesuvian eruption of 937% from the small base of 4.4 million recorded at the study's inception in 1987 -- Treadmills are the most successful exercise equipment ever. At nearly 46 million, (up only 5% in the past year) this activity seems near saturation; but strong links with health club expansion, aging demographics, and the continuing evolution of fitness holds the promise of a vast, perhaps inexhaustible pool of prospects. The phenomenal success of Treadmill Exercise can be traced to several roots; but the major attraction is the option to run or walk…and particularly, to walk as slowly as one likes. Conceived in another era, the timeless Treadmill has been somehow transported to the vanguard of Kinder/Gentler fitness.

Strength training is another ponderous giant which lately, never disappoints; year after year, it plods along, delivering uninterrupted single-digit growth. In 2003, there were a projected 51.6 million individuals in the U.S. who trained with some form of Free Weights -- an increase of 25% over 1998. Exactly 30 million used Weight/Resistance machines, up 33% from 1998.

Weight Training is no longer the exclusive province of hulking giants in dank muscle gyms. The activity has gone mainstream, and its most dramatic growth is traceable to the least likely demographics -- women and seniors. From 1987 - 2003, usage of Free Weights has grown from 22.6 million exercisers to 51.6 million -- an increase of 129%; but among women, the increase is an astounding 233%!

The growing popularity of lighter equipment -- Dumbbells and Hand Weights -- clearly (if counterintuitively) places Free Weight training at the center of Kinder/Gentler fitness.

The psychological dimensions of Kinder/Gentler, less taxing, less strenuous fitness are even more interesting than its physiology. In a "Comprehensive Study of American Attitudes toward Physical Fitness and Health Clubs", ASD has segmented the U.S. adult population into four groups: Consciousness I, II, III and IV. Consciousness IV is the "Hard-Core" group of 34.2 million devotees which has internalized fitness dogma and relentlessly converted to the active lifestyle. 45% are already Health Club members, while 18% work out at clubs but are not yet official inductees. 11% prefer Outdoors exercise, and 15% are Frequent Home Exercisers.

Consciousness III is the "Uninitiated Believer" -- stronghold of Kinder/Gentler fitness comprising over 60% of the population, said to be the "low-hanging" fruit -- ripe, easy pickings for recruiters and marketers seeking brand new converts. These acolytes need no further persuasion; a single spark will launch them into the fitness lifestyle.

"Curves for Women", the fastest growing retail franchise in American history, has provided this spark -- masterfully. With phenomenal, yet unceremonious growth -- this studio chain has grown from one outlet in 1992 to over 6,000 U.S. franchises in 2004 -- Curves has become the Mecca for Consciousness III, catering to unathletic, often overweight, sometimes older women, many of whom have never before joined a health club. A relatively inexpensive, (but intimate) bare-bones environment -- 30-minute "express" workouts, low-stress circuit training to music, no showers, lockers, or other amenities, the general absence of intimidating thongs, hardbodies, mirrors or other depressive influences -- has produced the ultimate democratization of fitness: eliminating virtually every excuse for not exercising, and making fitness available to everyone! (female, anyway...).

The "Curves" concept -- growing at the rate of 200 new outlets per month and frantically imitated by solo entrepreneurs and Health Club chains alike -- is not without detractors. Purists disdain the exercise regimen as "too easy", while others dismiss it as a mere fad.

ASD president Harvey Lauer feels that too much ink and energy is being wasted in a senseless debate over how many calories are burned in this "easier" workout routine. "Exercise physiologists miss the point completely" he says. "The true benefit of Curves is not caloric expenditure per se, but enhanced dieting stimulation. Women who do Express workouts are losing pounds and inches because they are also eating less. This newly found exercise-dieting mechanism functions like a perpetual motion machine -- one component driving the other."

On the other hand, business cynics fear the low franchise investments of $20,000 - $30,000 (and very high returns per square foot) impart an artificial boost…that Curves is more an entrepreneurial movement than a genuinely consumer-driven trend. Indeed, flameout is a possibility; but more likely, the "Express" workout is tracing an early arc of the fitness future.

The SUPERSTUDY® of Sports Participation was conducted in January 2004 and based on a nationally representative sample of 15,015 Americans over the age of 6, who were among 25,000 respondents targeted in a sample drawn from the consumer mail panel of NFO Worldwide. 103 sports and activities were measured along over 20 demographic, attitudinal and behavioral dimensions. Data were also collected on Health Club membership and other subjects pertinent to Physical Fitness. This annual tracking study has been conducted by ASD every year since 1987, and sponsored by the Sporting Goods Manufacturers Association of North Palm Beach, Florida and the International Health, Racquet & Sportsclub Association of Boston, Massachusetts. For more information, log onto www.americansportsdata.com.

* * *

U.S. PHYSICAL FITNESS TRENDS - SELECTED ACTIVITIES

Number of Participants (000)
1998-2003

	1998	2000	2001	2003	1-Year Change 2002-2003	5-Year Change 1998-2003
Pilates Training	n.a.	1,739	4,671	9,469	+103%	+445%[1]
Elliptical Motion Trainer	3,863	6,176	10,695	13,415	+25%	+247%
Yoga/Tai Chi	5,708	7,400	11,106	13,371	+20%	+134%
Recumbent Cycling	6,773	8,947	10,217	10,683	+5%	+58%
Weight/Resistance Machines	22,519	25,182	27,848	29,996	+8%	+33%
Free Weights (Net)	41,266	44,499	48,261	51,567	+7%	+25%
Treadmill Exercise	37,073	40,816	43,431	45,572	+5%	+23%
Home Gym Exercise	7,577	8,103	8,924	9,260	+4%[†]	+22%
Fitness Walking	36,395	36,207	37,987	37,945	+0%[†]	+4%
Running/Jogging	34,962	33,680	35,866	36,152	+1%[†]	+3%[†]
Fitness Biking	13,556	11,435	11,153	12,048	+8%[†]	-11%
Rowing Machine Exercise	7,485	6,229	7,092	6,484	-9%[†]	-13%
Stationary Cycling (Upright)	20,744	17,894	17,403	17,488	+1%[†]	-16%
Aerobics (Net)	21,017	17,326	16,046	16,451	+3%[†]	-22%
Stair-Climbing Machine Exercise	18,609	15,828	14,251	14,321	+1%[†]	-23%
Nordic Ski Machine Exercise	6,870	5,444	5,074	4,744	-7%[†]	-31%
Aerobic Rider Exercise	5,868	3,817	3,654	2,955	-19%	-50%
Health Club Membership (000)	29,483	32,808	36,289	39,405	+9%	+34%
Number of Health Clubs[2]	13,799	15,372	20,207	23,497	+16%	+70%

[1] = 3-year change   [2] = InfoUSA   [†] = not statistically significant at 95% Confidence Level

CHAPTER 13

A NEW FRONT IN THE WAR ON OBESITY

FOR IMMEDIATE RELEASE   July 13, 2004

* * *

<u>REALITY RESEARCH ROLLS OUT STATISTICS OF HUMAN POUNDAGE</u>

* * *

<u>Nearly 4 Million Americans Weigh Over 300 Pounds</u>

HARTSDALE, N.Y. -- A new front has been opened in the psychological war on obesity: publication of actual American bodyweight. Until now, the chief weapon in the informational war has been a polite abstraction -- "Body Mass Index", or BMI. But this simple, indispensable yet abstruse ratio of weight to height lacks the shock impact to ignite a national revolution.

The shelling has been noisy but light, with only vague generalities peppering the American consciousness -- such as "3 out of 5 Americans are overweight" or that "childhood obesity has nearly tripled in the last two decades." These are empty projectiles fired from heavy artillery, according to a new report by American Sports Data, Inc. (ASD).

In January 2004, a nationwide study of 12,094 adults (18+) -- sponsored by the International Health, Racquet &

Sportsclub Association (IHRSA) and conducted by ASD -- projected that 3.8 million Americans weighed more than 300 pounds. "Unless you're a well-proportioned 7-foot basketball player or a huge wrestler, that much body mass is hard to justify" said ASD president Harvey Lauer. "These are the eyebrow-raising figures we need to publicize -- not that the average woman has a BMI of 27.5, or that the rate of morbid obesity is 2.2%. Public health officials are logical, quantitative types who are scrupulous about data presentation -- but the art of communication is not necessarily part of their job description," he continued.

"People still aren't getting it. We need more visceral symbols of the obesity epidemic -- measures of the flesh that are vivid, graphic and powerful enough to galvanize a dangerously overweight population. Within the bounds of sensitivity, we need to hear more about pounds, inches, bodyfat percentages, sweating, panting, asthma, diabetes, heart attacks and premature death," concluded Lauer.

Men comprise 70% of the 300+ pound category, and also dominate a supermassive segment of 400,000 Americans who tip the scales at more than 400 pounds! 1 in 9 adult men carry more than 250 pounds, while 1 out of 6 women weighs in at over 200!

Adult males in the ASD study averaged 196 pounds; for women, the mean self-reported bodyweight was 163. In 1999 - 2000, the CDC-sponsored NHANES study, using mobile vans that criss-crossed the nation, physically weighed more than 4,000 adults (20+), calculating a mean of 177 -- similar to the later ASD finding of 179.

The current report on Obesity and Weight Control is derived from the Superstudy® of Sports Participation, conducted in January 2004 and based on a nationally representative sample of 15,015 people over the age of 6 who were among 25,000 respondents targeted in a sample drawn from the consumer mail panel of TNS-NFO. 103 sports and activities were measured along 20 demographic, attitudinal and behavioral dimensions. Data were also collected on health club membership, physical fitness, and weight control. This annual tracking study has been conducted by ASD every year since 1987. For more information log onto www.americansportsdata.com.

* * *

SELF-REPORTED BODYWEIGHT
U.S. ADULTS 18+
JANUARY 2004

	Male	Female
TOTAL SAMPLE	(6,324)	(5,770)
Population	101,651,000	109,463,000
	(%)	(%)
Under 100 pounds	-	1.0
101 - 124	1.1	13.2
125 - 149	7.9	27.5
150 - 174	21.6	22.5
175 - 199	27.9	14.5
200 - 224	19.6	8.8
225 - 249	9.7	3.7
250 - 299	8.0	3.9
300 - 349	1.6	0.7
350 - 399	0.7	0.2
400+	0.3	0.1
Not Reported	1.6	3.9
	100.0	100.0
Average Weight	196.0	162.8

Source: IHRSA/ASD Obesity-Weight Control Trend Report

CHAPTER 14

CONTRARIAN PHILOSOPHIES: FAT IS OKAY (ESPECIALLY IF YOU'RE FIT)

Every revolution begets a smaller counter-revolution, and the War on Obesity is no exception. One would imagine that an effort of such unquestioned altruism and nobility (to improve the psychological and physical health of a nation…even save millions of lives) would command a unanimity of public opinion. Naturally, one would be wrong.

The obesity epidemic in America is very well documented, and beyond the repetition of a few topline marquee numbers, I need not bore the reader with statistics found elsewhere in this book. Nearly two-thirds of Americans are overweight, a third obese. Child obesity has nearly tripled over the past 20 years, a frightful statistic which portends a truly calamitous public health future.

The aggregate impact of obesity -- in personal psychological suffering, physical deterioration and collectively, in the specter of a public health apocalypse -- is so immense as to justify an effort equal to or greater than that of the War on Smoking. But like its glorious predecessor, the anti-obesity crusade does not enjoy the categorical loyalty of Americans. There are five classes of objections.

Charlatans

A small subspecies of gadfly -- one has even written a book -- claims that the American obesity crisis is a gigantic hoax, perpetrated (of course!) by the Diet Industry. Demagogues claim that America is not only healthier, but living longer than ever -- and then speciously ask: "how can there be an obesity epidemic?" They conveniently fail to note that in the <u>absence</u> on an obesity epidemic U.S. public health achievements would be even greater!

Even worse, such opportunists deny the most abundant evidence of the crisis -- falsely claiming that Americans have gained only "a few pounds" over the last generation. This spurious argument is almost always cloaked in the legitimacy of the "fat and fit" philosophy.

BMI Naysayers

Another, less virulent breed takes issue with the BMI (Body Mass Index) calculation, a simple ratio of weight to height: weight in pounds, divided by height in inches, divided again by height in inches, then multiplied by 703. For adults, a BMI of under 25 is "normal"; 25-29.9 "overweight"; and 30+ "obese". BMI is an arbitrary (but extremely useful) gauge for the aggregate analysis of public health.

On an individual basis however, opponents of this guideline are correct in claiming that BMI is often incongruous with one's physical fitness and overall health; and also, that physical conditioning is far more important than bodyweight.

Victims

A large victimization subculture, led by a "victims' rights" advocacy embodying varying degrees of logic and authenticity, correctly focuses on societal abuse and intense suffering among overweight people. But these pleas for justice seldom mention individual responsibility for overeating. And there is a "fat and proud" movement, with a derivative contingent of "fat admirers" who prefer fat partners; but they are a tiny minority.

In general, people harbor a deep, primal revulsion to fatness, viewing morbid obesity as a hideous deformity, perceiving smaller deviations from the human ideal as proportionately less revolting -- but proof nonetheless, of indolence, indulgence and other violations of the Protestant Ethic.

Weight discrimination is one of the last bastions of social injustice, still awaiting the redress that has finally come to racial, female, gay and disabled minorities. But the movement functions most effectively as a shield -- not a sword wielded against the War on Obesity.

Righteously "Fat and Fit"

A fourth class of objectors has the greatest merit. They claim genetic predisposition to the overweight condition, and at the same time -- boast excellent health! Short, chunky and overweight -- but a healthy, avid runner and marathoner who has taken regular exercise for over 35 years -- Dr. Stephen Blair is the potential Poster Boy for this genre. Sporting a perfectly unacceptable Body Mass Index, Blair is senior scientific editor of the 1996 Report of the Surgeon General on Physical Activity and Health, and presumably one of the most fitness-conscious individuals in the land -- not a casualty of the great conflict.

There are countless others who evade the obesity dragnet, including sexy but outsized fashion models, and amateur athletes with prodigious indices of body mass, extremely graceful breed of overweight ballroom dancers. But these people are anomalies.

According to a 2002 national survey by American Sports Data, Inc. there were 39.5 million adults who described themselves as "considerably overweight". Of this number, only 4% (1.6 million) said they were in "excellent health"; 62% (24.3 million) described their health as "fair" or "poor".

With no pretensions to physiological analysis, ASD research can only offer several topline conclusions. First, there are relatively few adults in the U.S. who are <u>both</u> considerably <u>overweight</u> (by self-perception) <u>and very active</u> (250+ days of sports/exercise per year).

By these criteria, the "Fat and Fit" contingent of the U.S. population numbers 4.7 million -- only 2.3% of all adult Americans, but 12% of all people who dub themselves "considerably overweight". While not a startling number, this finding creates some awareness of a new subculture of "obese" exercisers -- and more importantly, an unlikely coterie of role models for a huge untapped fitness market.

The Insouciant Fat Majority

If overweight Americans now constitute a majority of the population, why change? This is by far the path of least resistance, and for some, an increasingly popular imprimatur of acceptability. It is also the most virulent strain of the "Fat is Okay" philosophy.

* * *

"CONSIDERABLY OVERWEIGHT"
BY SPORTS/EXERCISE PARTICIPATION
(39,521,000)

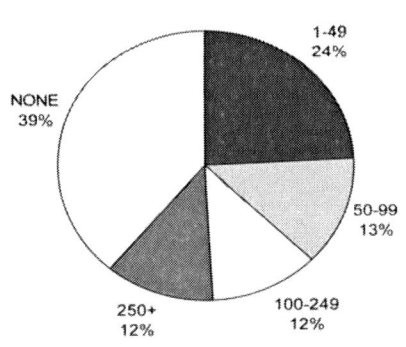

(DAYS PER YEAR)

- 1-49: 24%
- 50-99: 13%
- 100-249: 12%
- 250+: 12%
- NONE: 39%

Source: A Comprehensive Study of Consumer Attitudes Toward Physical Fitness and Health Clubs (2002).

CHAPTER 15

THE WEIGHT LOSS WARS: ADVANTAGE…HEALTH CLUBS

FOR IMMEDIATE RELEASE   July 26, 2004

* * *

*A MAJORITY OF AMERICANS
ARE TRYING TO LOSE WEIGHT*

* * *

*Dieting Works, But New Research Proves That
Frequent Health Club Exercise Is
The Most Successful Weight Loss Strategy*

HARTSDALE, N.Y. -- A clear majority of the U.S. population (65%) cares enough about its bodyweight to have taken some remedial action in the past year. But since the American desire to lose weight predates the War on Obesity, it is not clear if policy-makers, health officials, food companies, journalists, insurance companies and other weight loss warriors are finally beginning to move the behavioral needle.

In a nationwide study of 15,015 Americans conducted in January 2004 by American Sports Data, Inc. (ASD), nearly half the population (49%) said that at some point during 2003, they attempted to lose at least five pounds; another 16% indicated they had made an effort to maintain their weight. But only 20% of all people who tried to manage their weight felt that they were "very" or "extremely" successful -- even in the near term. These were findings of the IHRSA/ASD Obesity-Weight Control Report, derived from the SUPERSTUDY® of Sports Participation, an annual tracking study conducted every year since 1988.

Respondents in the nationally representative survey employed a number of weight loss techniques, but the great majority of those who tried to shed bodyweight (80%) kept it simple; they were just more careful about their eating habits. Nearly half (46%) worked out at home, while 38% opted for outdoors exercise. 20% placed their faith in a formal diet, and a similar number (19%) or 24.2 million, embraced health club exercise as a weight loss strategy. But a far greater number (43.2 million) used a gym for other reasons: cardio conditioning, muscle tone, flexibility, physical therapy, or to simply feel energized and refreshed -- incentives unrelated to weight loss.

For the sizeable minority of people who did use a gym for keeping trim, health club membership apparently confers certain advantages on the weight control process. Club members -- especially those who exercise frequently -- are far more likely than others to report successful weight loss experiences. 25% of all health club members who attempted to lose weight were "very" or "extremely" successful, compared with only 19% of hopefuls who did not attend a club. For members who exercised at their club at least 100 times throughout the year, the success rate soared to 30%.

"This finding", according to ASD president Harvey Lauer,

"is not a statistical fluke." In a 2002 study conducted with different methodology, frequent health club exercisers were highly successful in their quest to lose weight -- a result very nearly replicated by the present research.

"And not only is frequent health club exercise the most effective weight loss method, it confers physiological benefits unattainable through passive dieting, such as cardio conditioning and stamina, increased strength, muscle tone, bone density, and flexibility -- to name just a few."

Exactly how the gym experience inspires additional motivation or how the mechanics of club exercise enhance weight loss psychology is unclear, but health clubs may have several advantages. People who join clubs have the obvious benefit of positive reinforcement; they receive daily encouragement from other members and staff. But they also have the benefit of negative reinforcement -- the "invisible", unspoken, barely palpable peer pressure that is an equally powerful motivator. A more tangible incentive is the conscious need to get our money's worth; and for those who can afford one, the structure and discipline provided by a personal trainer offers a clear edge in the subliminal competition. Clubs also offer direct weight management assistance: weight loss programs, nutritional counseling, fitness evaluation, health education and other programs.

The study also found dieting an effective weight loss strategy: 26% of those who embraced a formal diet were very/extremely successful, while Outdoors and Home Exercise were not quite as effective, earning success rates of 21% and 19% respectively. Diet pills proved to be the very worst solution, satisfying only 12% of all weight loss aspirants.

In previous work, ASD has drawn a historic parallel between the present obesity epidemic and the war on smoking. Exactly 40 years after the landmark 1964 Surgeon General's Report, the incidence of adult smoking has been slashed dramatically, and -- the current blip in youth behavior notwithstanding -- may well be on the road to extinction. Some feel that in the War on Obesity, history will be repeated.

Others say that smoking cessation may have been easier. People simply had to stop smoking -- an indulgence found eventually to be deadly. In 2004 however, the U.S. population is not yet convinced that overeating can be lethal; nor can people just stop eating -- a powerful human instinct which happens also to provide one of life's greatest pleasures. But to level the playing field, overeaters have an antidote unavailable to smokers -- *physical activity*.

"Future medical historians", concludes Lauer, "will see this time as the beginning of an epic struggle, so what happens now is crucial. Although it's unquantifiable, we need to show the American public that the costs of obesity -- not just in deaths per year, but in aggregate physical, social and psychological suffering -- will exact a higher toll than the moribund practice of smoking."

The Weight Loss Wars

The current report on Obesity and Weight Control is derived from the Superstudy® of Sports Participation, conducted in January 2004 and based on a nationally representative sample of 15,015 people over the age of 6 who were among 25,000 respondents targeted in a sample drawn from the consumer mail panel of TNS-NFO. 103 sports and activities were measured along 20 demographic, attitudinal and behavioral dimensions. Data were also collected on health club membership, physical fitness, and weight control. This annual tracking study has been conducted by ASD every year since 1987. For more information log onto www.americansportsdata.com.

* * *

WEIGHT LOSS STRATEGIES
(LAST 12 MONTHS)

	TOTAL (000)	% OF PEOPLE ATTEMPTING WEIGHT LOSS (127,425,000)	% POPULATION 6+ (260,382,000)
Careful About Eating Habits	101,334	79.5	38.9
Home Exercise	59,106	46.4	22.7
Outdoors Exercise	48,551	38.1	18.6
Formal Diet	25,776	20.2	9.9
Health Club Exercise	24,155	19.0	9.3
Diet Pills (Over-the-Counter)	13,492	10.6	5.2
Prescription Diet Drugs	3,506	2.8	1.3
Laxatives	1,860	1.5	.7

* Multiple Responses Allowed

Source: IHRSA/ASD Obesity-Weight Control Report

WEIGHT LOSS EFFORT
"VERY/EXTREMELY SUCCESSFUL"
BY FREQUENCY OF ATTENDANCE
(HEALTH CLUB MEMBERS)
(%)

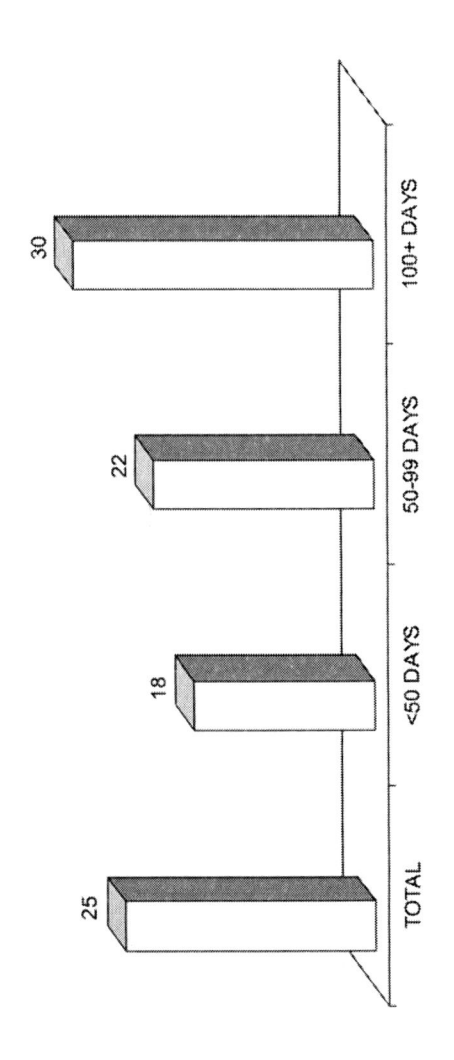

Category	%
TOTAL	25
<50 DAYS	18
50-99 DAYS	22
100+ DAYS	30

Source: IHRSA/ASD Obesity-Weight Control Report

WEIGHT LOSS EFFORT
(VERY/EXTREMELY SUCCESSFUL)
BY STRATEGY

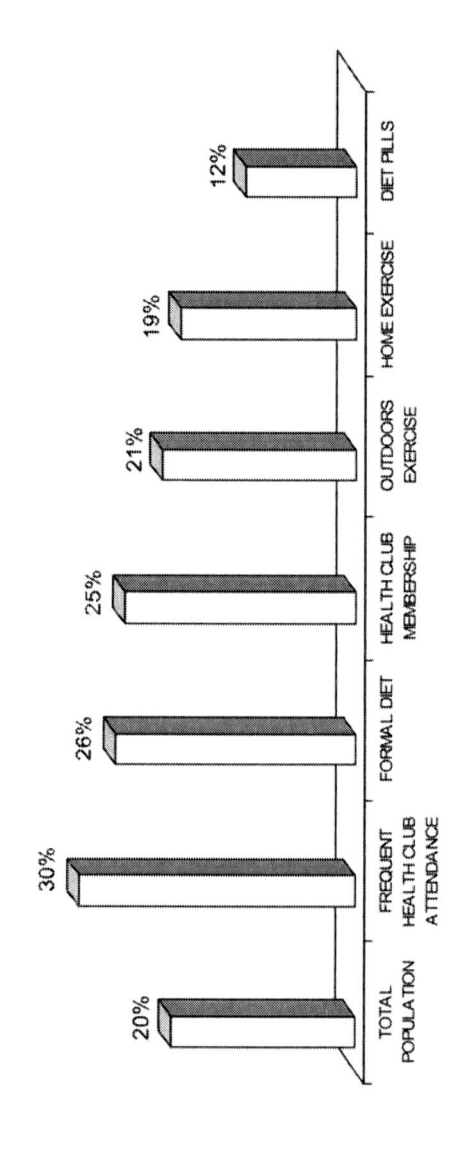

Strategy	Percentage
TOTAL POPULATION	20%
FREQUENT HEALTH CLUB ATTENDANCE	30%
FORMAL DIET	26%
HEALTH CLUB MEMBERSHIP	25%
OUTDOORS EXERCISE	21%
HOME EXERCISE	19%
DIET PILLS	12%

Source: IHRSA/ASD Obesity-Weight Control Report

CHAPTER 16

OLDER AMERICANS ARE TRANSFORMING LANDSCAPE OF PHYSICAL FITNESS

FOR IMMEDIATE RELEASE   April 12, 2005

* * *

A Quarter of 41.3 million Health Club Members are now over 55 as Seniors Drive Health Club Membership and Jump-Start a Resurgent Fitness Movement

HARTSDALE, N.Y. -- It languished for about a decade, but now the American fitness phenomenon is coming to life again, resuscitated by the least likely demographics -- "older" participants. From 1998 - 2004, the number of frequent fitness participants aged 55+ zoomed by 33%, compared with a growth rate of 13% for Baby Boomers aged 35-54, and *zero growth* for the "traditional" fitness participant aged 18-34. These were among the findings of the 18th annual SUPERSTUDY® of Sports Participation, conducted among 14,684 Americans nationwide in January 2005 by American Sports Data, Inc. (ASD).

25% of the nation's 41.3 million health club members are now over 55, the quintessential statistic that -- according to ASD president Harvey Lauer -- "represents not only a vast change in American attitudes and perceptions, but also an imminent restructuring of the health club and fitness industries, and most crucially -- the seed of monumental healthcare reform in the United States.

"The growth of senior fitness is the unifying theme that explains many of the changes we are seeing on the ground" he continued. It is no coincidence according to ASD, that the fastest-growing fitness activities in the U.S. are of the kinder-and-gentler variety that reflect older and disproportionately female age segments. Since 2000, Pilates has grown meteorically -- from just 1.7 million participants to 10.5 million in 2004 -- a quantum leap of 506%. Originally an exotic preserve for older women, Pilates continues to spill over into the mainstream -- inexorably declining in average participant age:

2000	43.6
2001	39.2
2002	35.1
2003	35.2
2004	33.7

With an average age of 38.5, Elliptical Motion Trainer exercise now claims 15.7 million fitness participants, an increase of 306% since 1998. After Treadmill Exercise and Stationary Cycling, this knee-friendly equipment is the third most popular form of cardio equipment exercise.

With participants averaging 38.2 years of age, the compound measurement of Yoga/Tai Chi has grown by 118% during 1998 - 2004. At 11.2 million participants, Recumbent Cycling, a particularly back-friendly exercise for older Americans, has grown 66% from 1998 - 2004. With an average age of 42.6, Recumbent Cycling is the third "oldest" fitness activity, surpassed in participant age only by Fitness Walking and Aquatics. Usage of Hand Weights and Dumbbells, still other examples of less taxing senior-friendly fitness, has increased by 29% and 34% respectively -- compared with a rise of only 13% in more strenuous Barbell lifting. People aged 55+ also constitute 25% of the 6.1 million Americans who paid for the services of a personal trainer in 2004.

Mature exercise enthusiasts are not merely playing havoc with abstract fitness statistics; they are rocking the foundations of fitness facilities across the U.S. Tremors of the senior shock wave are being felt throughout the health club industry, as YMCA/YWCA memberships increased substantially in 2004, along with "other" fitness facilities -- the survey classification which includes an exploding "Curves for Women" phenomenon and its Express Workout copycats. In the 2004 SUPERSTUDY® of Sports Participation, people over 55 comprised 35% of all memberships in "other" fitness facilities. Very strange bedfellows indeed, YMCA's and Express Workout clubs -- independent yet related phenomena that have dramatically impacted market share in the health club industry. "Curves", (the Mecca for older, out-of-shape women), and YMCA's, (the traditional haunt of aging exercisers), have unwittingly conspired to block the advance of high-end clubs.

Pricing trends are equally compelling. For the first time

since the inception of the research in 1988, average health club dues have dropped -- from $36.85 per month in 2003 to $33.90 in 2004: a startling 8% reversal but natural aftershock of the graying fitness revolution.

The massive influx of older exercisers has many roots, according to ASD:

1. Many of today's mature fitness participants were present at the genesis of the fitness revolution… these early converts made a lifetime commitment and never looked back. As the "pig" moved through the "python", those 30-somethings from the 1970's are now over 55.

2. Social norms have changed dramatically over the last 30-40 years. In the 1950's, the sight of an old man running through the streets in his underwear would have inspired our mothers or grandmothers to call the police; today, the image is commonplace. Fitness has achieved universal social acceptance (women can sweat and even grow muscles!) as exercise for seniors is widely mandated by medical professionals.

3. Increasingly, exercise is being prescribed for osteoporosis, hypertension, diabetes, heart disease and other maladies that afflict older populations.

4. The U.S. population is aging, and the average lifespan is increasing. Psychologically, there has been a 20-year shift in perceptions of age, and our expectation of vigorous life expectancy. A generation ago, 40 was "middle-aged", 50 was "old" and 60 was "dead". Today, 65 year-old children routinely care for 85 year-old parents.

5. Less taxing forms of exercise and equipment are being devised to accommodate an aging population…Kinder/Gentler fitness activities are enthusiastically promoted to attract and encourage senior participation. Yoga, Pilates, Recumbent Cycling, Treadmills, Fitness Walking, Aquatics, Hand Weights and last but least, Chair-Aerobics -- are all expressions of this megatrend.

The SUPERSTUDY® of Sports Participation was conducted in January 2005 and based on a nationally representative sample of 14,684 Americans over the age of 6, who were among 25,000 respondents targeted in a sample drawn from the consumer mail panel of NFO Worldwide. 103 sports and activities were measured along over 20 demographic, attitudinal and behavioral dimensions. Data were also collected on Health Club membership and other subjects pertinent to Physical Fitness. This annual tracking study has been conducted by ASD every year since 1987, and sponsored by the Sporting Goods Manufacturers Association of North Palm Beach, Florida and the International Health, Racquet & Sportsclub Association of Boston, Massachusetts. For more information, log onto www.americansportsdata.com.

* * *

FREQUENT FITNESS PARTICIPATION*
By Age Group
(000)

	1998	2003	2004	1-Year Change 2003-2004	6-Year Change 1998-2004
6-11	2,261	1,829	1,965	+ 7.4%[†]	- 13%[†]
12-17	5,733	5,153	5,182	+ 0.6%[†]	- 9%[†]
18-34	13,511	14,389	13,533	- 6%[†]	0
35-54	17,912	19,799	20,258	+ 2%	+13%
55+	11,886	13,708	15,751	+15%	+33%
	51,303	54,878	56,689	+ 3%	+11%

* at least 100 times in any single fitness activity

[†] not statistically significant at 95% Confidence Level

Older Americans Drive Physical Fitness

U.S. PHYSICAL FITNESS TRENDS - SELECTED ACTIVITIES

Number of Participants (000)

	1998	2003	2004	1-Year Change 2003-2004	6-Year Change 1998-2004
Pilates Training	n.a.	9,469	10,541	+11%	+506%[1]
Elliptical Motion Trainer	3,863	13,415	15,678	+17%	+306%
Yoga/Tai Chi	5,708	13,371	12,414	- 7%	+118%
Recumbent Cycling	6,773	10,683	11,227	+ 5%(†)	+ 66%
Weight/Resistance Machines	22,519	29,996	30,903	+ 3%(†)	+ 37%
Dumbbells	23,414	30,549	31,415	+ 3%(†)	+ 34%
Hand Weights	23,325	29,720	30,143	+ 1%(†)	+ 29%
Treadmill Exercise	37,073	45,572	47,463	+ 4%	+ 28%
Home Gym Exercise	7,577	9,260	9,347	+ 1%(†)	+ 23%
Barbells	21,263	25,645	24,103	- 6%	+ 13%
Fitness Walking	36,395	37,945	40,299	+ 6%	+ 11%
Running/Jogging	34,962	36,152	37,310	+ 3%(†)	+ 7%
Rowing Machine Exercise	7,485	6,484	7,303	+ 13%	- 2%(†)
Stationary Cycling (Upright)	20,744	17,488	17,889	+ 2%(†)	- 14%
Aerobics (Net)	21,017	16,451	15,767	+ 4%(†)	- 25%
Outdoor Fitness Biking	13,556	12,048	10,210	- 15%	- 25%
Stair-Climbing Machine Exercise	18,609	14,321	13,300	- 7%(†)	- 29%
Nordic Ski Machine Exercise	6,870	4,744	4,155	- 12%(†)	- 40%
Aerobic Rider Exercise	5,868	2,955	2,468	- 17%(†)	- 58%
Health Club Membership (000)	29,483	39,405	41,338	+ 5%	+ 40%
Frequent Fitness Participants (100+ Days)	51,303	54,878	56,689	+ 3%	+ 11%
Personal Trainer Usage	4,021	5,288	6,154	+ 16%	+ 53%

[1] = 4-year change   (†) = not statistically significant at 95% Confidence Level

- 153 -

CHAPTER 17

PHYSICAL FITNESS: A THUMBNAIL HISTORY

If we ignore the ancient Greeks, the rest of antiquity, and also the next couple of thousand years, we can trace physical fitness to the Industrial Revolution -- the epochal transformation from vigorous agrarian life in the countryside to a more sedentary existence in the bigger cities of Europe. Arguably, the need for recreational exercise was first manifest in 1847 when Hippolyte Triat, a former Vaudevillian strongman, established the first health club (gymnasium) in Paris. In the same decade, the YMCA movement was begun in England by Sir George Windship. This new conception embodied "Muscular Christianity" -- a curious hybrid of spiritual and physical well-being.

Muscular Christianity and the YMCA movement would eventually migrate to America, but not before the evangelism of George Barker Windship -- a puny Harvard undergraduate -- who (not unlike Teddy Roosevelt) sought to remedy his diminutive physique through gymnastics and weight training. Windship is the reputed father of American strength training -- the dominant form of physical fitness for the next century.

At the end of the 19th century, physical education -- thoroughly intertwined with character building -- was introduced into American school systems. Both phenomena were to suffer long, tragic declines in the 20th century.

1910 marked the invention of the barbell, and the 1920's witnessed the golden age of the Vaudevillian strongman. Inaugurated in 1927, a small strip of California shoreline became known as "Muscle Beach" -- the Mecca of American bodybuilding. In the late 1930's and early 1940's, two of its graduates, Jack LaLanne and Vic Tanny, inaugurated the first weight-lifting club chains in the world, with Joe Gold, a later icon who in 1964 founded an empire that numbered over 600 clubs by the year 2000. But until the true <u>cardio</u> fitness revolution of the 1970's (which engaged a significant percentage of the American population) strength-training -- although synonymous with physical fitness -- <u>was not a mass phenomenon</u>. Although many were clean, well-lit facilities with amenities, health clubs of the day were perceived as dark, dank, "sweat and spit" dungeons -- the exclusive province of hulking male bodybuilders. Thongs would come much later.

Fitness and the New Focus on "Self"

Because it transcended mere physical exercise, the modern American fitness movement represents one of the most profound cultural changes of the 20th century. The trend toward improved health and fitness is a component of the larger shift in our national consciousness termed by social scientist Daniel Yankelovich the "Search for Self-Fulfillment". It too emerged from the turbulent 1960's counterculture, and is best depicted by its absence, when the group and its authority -- not the individual -- was the building block of society.

It is difficult to imagine a time when people rarely questioned the authority and wisdom of parents, teachers, policemen, clergymen

A Thumbnail History of Physical Fitness

or civil defense wardens; when we naively believed everything in print, and with childish deference, exempted public officials (and most other successful people) from the vices and failings that could afflict only "us". Blind obedience and groupthink were not fertile grounds for self-development.

Bookstores of the 1940's and 1950's did not yet have books on self-help -- let alone entire departments dedicated to self-improvement. Feeling "a little out of sorts" hardly justified regular visits to a psychiatrist; concern for personal health and well-being had not yet grown to a national obsession, and people were certainly not about to punish themselves with inconvenience, physical pain or the discomfort of regular exercise -- even if it meant better health and a heightened sense of well-being. The counterculture had little to do with physical fitness. Indeed, those old enough to remember are left with deafening, smoke-filled images that were by any reckoning, quite alien to improved health or fitness. For most hippies, the "Me-Generation" of the 1970's -- when people would truly embrace self-fulfillment -- was the gift of a distant future.

Until the 1970's, the small percentage of fitness participants in the U.S. were essentially <u>goal-oriented</u>. A handful may have been driven by the pure benefits of exercise, but most engaged in structured fitness activities for specific reasons: sports training, stamina building, muscle tone, or in rare cases, even recreational enjoyment. Younger participants were invariably students in the more serious P.E. classes of the day.

Then came the Fitness revolution. Not only was it several orders of magnitude larger than anything that came before, the Fitness boom of the 1970's was also <u>self-oriented</u>. People were drawn to the new cardio revolution for the nebulous, unspecific goal of self-improvement -- and to its new iconography. Nylon running suits worn as everyday streetwear became symbolic of a superior breed which exercised for not only traditional reasons -- but for the new, higher values of self-expression and self-fulfillment. A bicycle clip on the right pant leg became an ecological status symbol, no less a socio-political statement than Granny Glasses, Perrier or the ritualistic consumption of Crunchy Granola.

Planted in the 1960's, the value of "self" finally took root and spilled over into the general population during the 1970's. Self-improvement was the megatrend that began to sweep the nation, with concern for personal health a component trend, and physical fitness a sub-trend. Launched by Frank Shorter's Marathon victory in the 1972 Olympics, the original New York City Marathon in Central Park and Jim Fixx's 1977 landmark book -- the Running Boom (eclipsing a Cycling boomlet) became spearhead of the Fitness Revolution. More precisely, it eclipsed a cycling boomlet and heralded the <u>cardio</u> Fitness Revolution.

Not coincidentally, the exercise boom -- perfectly synchronized with a Health Food craze, a psychological Self-Help genre, a cult of Self-Expression and an unprecedented spate of Mind/Body improvements -- simultaneously announced the birth of the Fitness Revolution. It may have been a descendent of the 1960's counterculture, but the new Health and Fitness consciousness was a child of the 1970's "Me-Generation".

A Thumbnail History of Physical Fitness

There will always be a question about the role of Tennis in the early Fitness boom. With over 30 million players in 1974, Tennis was king. Today, most people play Tennis for recreational enjoyment (71% according to a 1996 study by American Sports Data, Inc.) while only 26% are motivated by physical fitness. The great Tennis boom of the early 1970's was to at least some degree fitness-inspired; but the exact proportions are lost to prehistory. Ironically, fitness would be the undoing of Tennis; by 2004, the sport had withered to 18.3 million players.

The proto-Health Club of the 1970's was a Racquet club dominated by Tennis courts (and later Racquetball) with a few Stationary Bikes and Rowing Machines in the corner. But during the early 1980's the balance would shift away from Racquet sports toward Aerobics classes, new types of cardio and Weight equipment. Inevitably, Health Clubs would evolve into the lavish multi-purpose Fitness palaces of the 1990's.

The modern cardio fitness movement proceeded through four distinct phases, of which the Running boom was first. By the early 1980's, Running had inspired a second wave of high-impact or otherwise strenuous fitness activities such as Aerobics, Fitness Biking and the Triathlon. The late 1980's witnessed a third generation of potentially easier, less stressful low-impact exercise opportunities such as Fitness Walking, Soft Aerobics, Stationary Cycling and Treadmill Exercise -- activities less threatening and more user-friendly to a large, sedentary element of the population which may have been intimidated by earlier "hard-core" fitness trends. Consequently, this third wave of fitness boom -- represented by overweight, unathletic, (and, in many cases, older) segments of the population -- was the real revolution, because it made fitness available to everyone.

By 1990, there were 51.5 million frequent fitness participants in the U.S. -- a quantum leap from the (presumed) near-zero baseline of the 1950's. But it marked the end of a long upward trajectory, and the beginning of a plateau that would span more than a decade. Paradoxically -- undoubtedly aided by a failure of self-motivation among many fitness enthusiasts -- Health Club membership continued to grow throughout the 1990's.

Phase four of the Fitness Revolution, "Kinder/Gentler Fitness" -- begun in the late 1990's and early New Millennium -- is bolstering the megatrend; in 2004, 25% of the nation's 41.3 million Health Club members were over 55 years of age. Senior fitness is the unifying theme of many growth measurements, including Pilates, Yoga, Treadmill Exercise, Hand-Weights, Recumbent Stationary Cycling, Health Club and YMCA membership, not to mention "Curves for Women" -- the most prolific franchise in American history, heralding the ultimate democratization of fitness. Still, in 2004, there were only 56.7 million frequent participants, a population incidence of 21.6% -- down from 23.2% in 1990.

Healthy Lifestyle Incentives: The Missing Motivational Link?
Despite the current obesity epidemic -- and a lukewarm behavioral record since 1990 -- our collective fitness-consciousness is highly evolved and surprisingly strong. In three separate tracking studies since 1996, ASD has documented that while only 20% of the population are frequent exercisers, many more

A Thumbnail History of Physical Fitness

(around 80% of all adults) are at some level, persuaded of its virtues; most in fact, think they should exercise more. To firm up a weakening resolve, millions of Americans -- in the face of an overall lackluster fitness movement -- are flocking to Health Clubs and Personal Trainers. A statistic worth repeating is that health club membership in the U.S. now stands at 41.3 million -- dwarfing the 1987 count of 17.4 million by 138%. In 2004, 6.2 million Americans paid for the services of a Personal Trainer -- up 55% since 1999.

Physical fitness activity, as it relates to bodyweight, is a complex issue; but it plays directly into the hands of incentivization. For the 1990's, we have a slight erosion of sports/fitness behavior, rising obesity levels, but at the same time, <u>a major plea for help</u> -- evidenced by skyrocketing Health Club and Personal Trainer usage. Americans are very fitness-conscious, but struggle to overcome a perennial lack of discipline; fitness behavior simply lags enlightened attitudes. In any event, the nation is primed: incentives and subsidies which promote healthier living could easily shape the future of public health.

* * *

CHAPTER 18

WAVE OF THE FUTURE:
THE SUBSIDIZATION OF PHYSICAL FITNESS
(CLUB BUSINESS INTERNATIONAL -- MARCH 2006)

I have been asked to prophesy the future of the Health Club industry over the next 25 years. This is not a daunting task, because during my charter membership in the World Future Society back in 1967, I learned that the long-term future is a lot easier to forecast than the short-term. That shibboleth underlies my favorite press quote: "By the year 2050, all able-bodied Americans will exercise; those who do not will be pariahs -- like people who didn't brush their teeth everyday back in 2006".

Predictions for the year 2030 are just as easy, and there are many to choose from: the ultimate democratization of fitness (everyone does it); the dominance of Kinder/Gentler (Senior) exercise; undreamed-of advances in health club technology; a brave new world of "magic pills" transcending the need for diet or exercise (not a good thing); a collective slimming of the American Waistline (science-fiction indeed!) and a host of others.

But one edifice of the future towers majestically above all others. It is visible through only the most powerful and extraordinary field glasses -- ones capable of peering into the future, as well as the distant past. The transforming event of the next 25 years: a universal subsidization of physical fitness.

The Old Medical Paradigm: Remedial Healthcare

For thousands of years, the history of medicine has been remedial and therapeutic. The art of healing was invoked only <u>after</u> the patient became ill, injured, disabled or otherwise indisposed. Traditionally, professional medicine was required to repair broken bodies, cure diseases or comfort those who could not be cured or restored. It was easy for this paradigm to reign for so long, because as late as the mid-twentieth century, people defined health in very narrow terms. Health was purely a physical phenomenon and good health simply meant the absence of disease; it was also the responsibility of doctors -- not individuals.

This is not to diminish the exemplary history of public health, which through immunization, nutrition, sanitary reform and scientific advancement, numbers -- among its many other conquests -- the scourges of smallpox, typhus, malaria, cholera, tuberculosis and polio. But just a tiny percentage of traditional medicine was of the preventive variety…and this was <u>passive preventive healthcare</u> facilitated by scientific progress, improvement of infrastructure and other factors which had nothing to do with the individual.

The modern era of <u>active preventive healthcare</u>, as it pertains to active lifestyle behavior by the individual -- began in 1964 with the landmark report of the Surgeon General on Smoking.

Several decades ago came a values shift of epic proportions. Beyond its traditional meaning, the definition of health was expanded to include the psychological realm; the idea of good health evolved to a higher state of mental, as well as physical well-being. In addition to this basic redefinition came another monumental change in medical philosophy: good health became the partial responsibility of the <u>individual</u> -- not just the medical profession. Thus, in large part, was born the concept of incentivized personal healthcare through healthier living, and subsequently, a platform of new preventive strategies which are just now being embraced -- somewhat half-heartedly -- by health insurers, employers and governmental policymakers. This new era is in its infancy.

Decision-makers are finally realizing that healthier people make more productive employees, file fewer insurance claims and make fewer demands on already-strapped government funding. Policymakers are being prodded toward subsidized preventive healthcare…but in many cases, their reluctant homage to this revolutionary concept takes the form of lip-service.

Nearly two-thirds of the nation is overweight, as 4 million Americans now tip the scales at more than 300 pounds. The average adult female weighs in at 165, with men about to burst through a national mean bodyweight of 200 pounds. Despite a quantum leap in our health and fitness consciousness over the past several decades, 4 out of 5 people are still relatively inactive: A combination of poor eating habits and physical inactivity has produced a grotesque sideshow in which the term "Ugly American" -- formerly a political epithet -- is invested with a new, equally disturbing symbolism.

Evolutionary social change is rarely announced by headlines, parades, crashing cymbals or other fanfare. But a silent and momentous transformation is now underway, as ordinary Americans, with the help of HMO's, insurers, corporations and government agencies, are being given the opportunity to quietly take control of their personal health, to live longer, healthier, more enjoyable lives, and as a by-product -- help tame a wildly out-of-control healthcare system.

This unprecedented paradigm shift -- from remedial to preventive healthcare -- represents a massive change in American attitudes and public policy which allows the individual -- through personal behavior modification encouraging healthier lifestyles -- to share the responsibility for good health with the medical profession. A host of personal incentives, underwritten by major policy changes, are being created to navigate this sea change in medical philosophy.

The Psychology of Entitlement
Two generations ago, the idea that people are "entitled" to certain things "for nothing" was embraced by only a handful of wild-eyed radicals; but eventually, that fluffy radical notion became the bedrock of mainstream psychology. No longer dirty words whispered by crypto-Marxists, "subsidization" and "entitlement programs" were elevated to commonplace terms in the lexicon. Just as luxuries evolved into necessities (the automobile, for example) good health and its closest surrogates (healthcare and health insurance) were eventually sanctified as inalienable human rights.

By the 1970's, it had become an unquestioned principle imbued with moral urgency. Most Americans believed that the government had a legal obligation to help the needy -- to fulfill certain basic human needs -- regardless of the individual's ability to pay for those services. With roots in the 1960's counterculture, this belief system, dubbed "psychology of entitlement", was popularized by social theorist Daniel Yankelovich more than a quarter-century ago.

The spirit of entitlement -- perhaps inaptly named -- is very much alive in 2005. Health insurance is of course, part of today's compensation package; but this is only a technicality. Americans regard healthcare as a basic necessity and right...with only a small step remaining to the subsidization of gym memberships, diet plans, nutritional supplements, and many other preventive healthcare measures.

Physical Fitness will soon be a standard health benefit, even an entitlement.

Americans Favor Subsidized Fitness

Health is a cherished American value, and the endless torrent of research linking exercise with better health is almost, but not quite, tedious. People believe in the subsidization of preventive healthcare -- partly from a lingering sense of entitlement, but also because they lack self-discipline and require the additional motivation of financial incentives. According to a January 2004 survey conducted for IHRSA by Ketchum Global Research Network, Americans strongly support action by health insurance providers, employers and government to promote physical fitness and a healthy lifestyle. While independent research sources have come to the triangulated conclusion that only 1 out of 5 people exercise on a regular basis, the IHRSA study found that…

- Three-fourths of Americans (77%) would be "very" or "somewhat" likely to exercise if they paid a lower health insurance premium;

- 70% believe that patients should be reimbursed for physician-prescribed fitness/exercise programs;

- Eight in ten Americans (82%) say they would exercise regularly if their employer subsidized Health Club memberships;

- Six out of ten (61%) believe that Congress should do more to promote physical activity and prevent obesity.

Healthy Lifestyle Incentives: A Ranking of Consumer Preferences
According to a 2002 study conducted for IHRSA by American Sports Data, Inc., consumers have a clear notion of which subsidized benefits they prefer. The following are the benefits they'd like, ranked by order of preference:

1. Full Medical Checkup
2. Exercise classes
3. A Health Club membership
4. Nutritional counseling
5. Smoking cessation program
6. Weight-control program (i.e. Weight Watchers)
7. Medical care for sports/exercise injuries
8. Other preventive care (chiropractic, massage therapy, etc.)
9. Stress-reduction program (i.e. Yoga, Biofeedback, etc.)
10. Home exercise equipment
11. Nutritional supplements (vitamins/health foods)
12. Services of a personal trainer
13. Fitness monitoring devices (heart rate monitor, pedometer, running log, etc.)

14. Athletic footwear/apparel
15. Home exercise videos
16. Special diet product

* Prescription drugs for obesity (not ranked)
* Surgery for obesity (not ranked)

Pioneers of Prevention

Most HMO's will pay for medically-based preventive healthcare such as screenings and vaccinations, and until recently, the subsidization of healthy lifestyles was still too new, radical or "frivolous" to merit serious consideration. Smoking is still a vice, undeserving of special preventive attention. To the Old Guard, physical fitness activities are still "recreational pursuits"; and despite the well-documented obesity epidemic, there are some reactionary forces that at best, view subsidized weight control programs as concessions to the self-indulgent; at worst, simply cosmetic and narcissistic.

Lacking the imprimatur of medical legitimacy, the incentivization of healthy lifestyle behavior does not yet command the urgency (and dollars) accorded to acute healthcare, disease management, or even the more compelling medical variants of preventive healthcare. But the recent Medicare sanction of obesity as a bona fide "disease" could change everything.

Even prior to the new ruling, major institutions (particularly in the private sector) had overcome major obstacles. Among them:

- In July 2004, Medicare redefined obesity as an <u>illness</u>, a massive policy change that may allow millions of Americans to make medical claims for prescription drugs, counseling, diet programs and even surgery related to obesity. In that private insurers often follow the lead of Medicare, the decision is monumental. But the present context of obesity is "remedial" -- not "preventive".

- In March 2004, then-U.S. Secretary of Health and Human Services Tommy G. Thompson urged Congress to offer tax credits to people who lose weight, and exhorted insurance companies to offer reduced premiums to those who shed poundage permanently.

- In August 2005, physician-prescribed remedial (not preventive) exercise programs for specific health issues were allowed by the IRS as "qualified medical expenses".

- To curb runaway Medicaid costs, the state of Michigan, in September 2005, announced a plan to incentivize healthy behaviors such as smoking cessation, maintaining doctor's appointments and weight control.

- Under a 2005 agreement reached between officials of King County in the state of Washington, county workers will earn points for healthier living and better disease management -- including smoking cessation, seat belt usage, diabetes monitoring and cholesterol screening.

- The 2004 Benefits Survey conducted by the <u>Society for Human Resource Management</u> revealed that 30% of companies subsidize fitness center membership, while 50% of large companies (500+ employees) subsidize employee weight loss programs. Industries most likely to subsidize fitness centers: Government (39%), Manufacturing (39%), Health (36%), Technology (32%), Retail (31%).

- <u>Oxford Health Plan</u> offers a $200 rebate (check mailed directly to policyholders) who prove that they have attend-

The Subsidization of Physical Fitness

ed a health club at least 50 times in the past 6 months. Oxford also offers a 10% - 40% discount on a wide array of healthy lifestyle expenditures, including…
    …exercise equipment
    …diabetic products
    …weight loss programs
    …fitness publications
    …spa services
    …eyewear
    …Yoga and Pilates programs

- PacifiCare Health Systems offers prizes to members who enroll in and maintain a disease management or preventive healthcare behavior regimen.

- Aetna provides a discount on health club memberships for its dental and medical participants -- but not for mere attendance, without a membership.

- Participants in a five year-old Destiny Health program are awarded points for taking a CPR class, starting an exercise program, losing 10 pounds in 6 months, checking their cholesterol level, and using the Internet to look up information.

- HIP Health Plan of New York members receive up to a 30% discount on acupuncture, massage, relaxation, fitness and related services.

Obstacles to Progress

Giving birth is never easy, and evolution is never entirely cooperative; for HMO's sponsoring HEALTHIER PEOPLE programs, most efforts seem nominal. Programs have been written, rebates disbursed to all who have become aware of healthier living benefits, but surprisingly -- many policyholders remain uninformed that such benefits exist! To a large degree, healthy lifestyle incentives -- from both insurers and corporations -- have been a well-kept secret. In 2004, only 4% of all IHRSA clubs had an HMO/Insurance affiliation.

Indifference to inspired policymaking must be underwritten by powerful, but flawed logic. To date, neither insurers nor employers can quantify the ROI for healthier lifestyle programs because <u>research methodology</u> that even purports to weigh the savings of reduced insurance claims against the cost of rebates or premium reductions <u>does not yet exist</u>. Consequently -- especially in troubled times -- policyholder rebates or credits (lacking ROI sanctification) are seen as pure bottom-line erosion, without payback. So despite the noble birth of such programs, insurers and employers have little motivation to encourage such an unquantifiable abstraction. And health insurance providers -- like their close cousins in most other insurance businesses -- are inherently conservative.

Health clubs and other end-providers of healthy lifestyle services may also have limited incentives to popularize these insurance benefits because the consumer -- not the club -- is often the direct beneficiary of reduced premiums. But clubs should be thinking about recruitment and retention…about how much easier rejoining might be for a member who <u>knows</u> that a $200 insurance rebate (or an even heftier percentage of dues) awaits him or her…or about how much easier it might be to sell a new member with such a huge incentive.

The Subsidization of Physical Fitness

The Coming Importance of Fitness Assessment

However distant the objective -- and no matter how few observers are equipped with the requisite field glasses -- our first baby steps are invariably borne of simple bottom-line common sense, and have a certain innocence; people are rewarded for <u>good intentions</u>, such as health club membership, participating in diet programs, even the simple act of buying a book on nutrition -- <u>not on measured results or outcomes</u>. This however, is a natural beginning; more logical, effective schemes (based on actual health improvement) will come later.

Eventually, those who pay the bills (e.g. HMO's) will grow weary of blanket rebates without calibrated returns, and rewards to policy-holders will transition to measurable criteria: weight and bodyfat reduction, improved cholesterol levels, heart rates, blood pressure and other quantifiable indicators of progress. At this inevitable stage, the once-insignificant Health Club profit center of FITNESS ASSESSMENT will be perfectly positioned to become supreme arbiter of improved health -- <u>for both members and outside non-members</u> who will now need to qualify for the new, more stringent rebate based on <u>OUTCOMES</u> of healthier living.

* * *

TWELVE METHODS OF SUBSIDIZING HEALTH CLUB MEMBERSHIP
(PRESENT AND FUTURE)

1. Employer has <u>on-site</u> facility
2. Employer pays for <u>outside</u> club
3. Employer pays health insurance that:
   …covers health club membership
   …issues premium credits to employer
   …issues rebates to employer
4. HMO/Insurance Plan issues <u>rebates</u> directly to policy-holder
5. HMO/Insurance Plan issues insurance premium credits
6. HMO/Insurer reimburses club for policyholder attendance/progress
7. Government "covers" preventive healthcare expenses (Traditional Model -- Medicare/other third party pays health club)
8. Government gives individual taxpayers <u>partial</u> reimbursement by allowing health club membership deduction on 1040 Schedule A
9. Government gives individual taxpayers <u>full</u> reimbursement by allowing health club membership tax credit (as a deduction for net tax bill) on 1040. (Similar to Child Care Credit)
10. Government allows corporate taxpayers a deduction on Form 1120 for dues payments to outside clubs on behalf of employees; beneficiaries (employees) are exempt from reporting such benefits as income
11. Free fitness facility provided by government agency
12. Health Club Dues Payment as an option selected from a <u>Consumer-Driven Health Plan</u>

The Subsidization of Physical Fitness

PREVENTIVE HEALTHCARE

SOCIETAL

- Air Pollution
- Water Pollution
- Sanitation
- Food Regulation
- Drug Approval
- Worksite Safety
- Toxic Waste Disposal
- Community Protection
- Product Safety
- Gun Control
- Sports Safety Rules
- Anti-Smoking Restrictions
- Seat-Belt Legislation
- Speed Limits
- School Cafeteria Guidelines
- IRS Rulings (Healthy Living Deductions)
- Medicare Legislation
- Maternity Care
- Prenatal Care
- Public Health Infrastructure
- Other Infrastructure

PERSONAL

PASSIVE

- Full Medical Checkups
- Breast Exams
- Mammography
- Pap Tests
- PSA Screening
- HIV Testing
- Cholesterol Check
- Blood Pressure Monitoring
- Colorectal Cancer Screening
- Diabetes Screening
- Weight Checks
- Vision, Hearing, Balance Evaluations
- Testicular Exams
- Glaucoma Screening
- Transmittable Disease Screenings

ACTIVE

MEDICAL SOLUTIONS/DRUGS

- Cholesterol Medication
- Blood Pressure Medication
- Prescription Diet Pills
- Gastro Bypass Surgery
- Sleep Disorder Therapy
- Vaccinations:
  - Influenza
  - Pneumonia
  - Rubella
  - Tetanus
  - Hepatitis
  - Chicken Pox

LIFESTYLE CHANGES

- Home Exercise
- Outdoors Exercise
- Health Club Exercise
- Dieting
- Eating Habits
- Smoking Cessation
- Alcohol Consumption
- Stress Reduction
- Sexual Behavior
- Substance Abuse
- Dental Care
- Seat-Belt Use
- Personal Safety
- Worksite Behavior

PART THREE:

SPORTS PARTICIPATION

CHAPTER 19

"EXTREME SPORTS" BONANZA

FOR IMMEDIATE RELEASE   April 1, 2001

* * *

National Tracking Study Unveils a Mixed Year, As Gains in Some Contemporary Activities May Be at the Expense of Traditional American Sports and Pastimes

* * *

Health Clubs and Personal Trainers Motivate Reluctant Exercisers, Buoying Fitness Sector

HARTSDALE, N.Y. -- True to form, Snowboarding, Skateboarding and Wakeboarding -- three of the so-called "Extreme" or "Millennial" sports -- were the fastest growing in the U.S. during the first year of the New Millennium. This was according to the 14th annual Superstudy® of Sports Participation, conducted in January, 2001 by American Sports Data, Inc. among 14,772 Americans nationwide.

During the year 2000, Snowboarding -- once the unwanted stepchild of the ski slopes -- skyrocketed by 51% to 7.2 million participants. The kindred activities of Skateboarding and Wakeboarding surged by 49% and 32% respectively, giving this sub-genre of "board" sports a clean sweep of the top three growth positions. Three other "Alternative Sports" earned a top ten rating. In a statistical tie, Surfing and Artificial Wall Climbing captured sixth place, both leaping by 26% over 1999 measurements. With 2 million participants and an 18% growth rate, Snowshoeing secured tenth position.

These emerging sports (variously dubbed "Millennial", "Alternative", or "New Age") are the province of Generation Y males, and -- depending on the commentator -- also include activities such as Wall-Climbing, Surfing, Paintball, Mountain Biking, BMX, In-Line Skating and Snowshoeing. The common defining feature of Extreme sports is the adrenaline-rush produced by the thrill and excitement of being "on the edge".

In-Line Skating, progenitor of the Extreme sports category, first appeared in the late 1980's, and then grew meteorically -- to a peak of 32 million participants in 1998. After reaching this saturation point, the skating population receded by 13% in 1999 to 27.9 million, and based on dwindling product sales, seemed destined to slide even further. But in the year 2000, presumably on the coattails of its offspring, this original Extreme sport stabilized at 29 million -- a statistically insignificant increase of 4% over 1999. Although it attracted 13.9 million youthful participants (average age 13.2) in 2000, the trendy activity of Scooter Riding (80% were newcomers) did not, as some industry analysts feared, hasten the decline of In-Line Skating.

In cooperation with the Extreme trend, an abundance of snow in many regions practically assured a dominant rating for Snowboarding. And so obliging was the weather that every single snow sport -- Extreme or otherwise -- enjoyed growth during 2000. The number of people who operated a Snowmobile jumped 28%, to 7 million, while the ranks of those who engaged in Snowshoeing and Cross-Country Skiing swelled respectively by 18% and 16%. Downhill Skiing was a lesser beneficiary, advancing only 6% for the year -- but the result did not achieve statistical significance.

But the blessings of Extreme sports may come at a price no less dear than that of American traditions. For the year 2000, the survey found 10.9 million Baseball players in the U.S. -- 10% fewer than in 1999 and a 28% deficit from 1987. Basketball declined by 5% in the past year and 17% from its 1997 peak. Since 1987, Softball and Volleyball have plunged by 37% and 36% respectively, with Touch Football falling a little less precipitously -- by 24%. On the positive side of the ledger, Soccer remained flat (+1%), while Fast-Pitch Softball and Tackle Football advanced by 18% and 15% respectively. But since the latter two measurements barely attained statistical significance, they merit further observation, said Lauer.

According to ASD president Harvey Lauer, "traditional team sports such as Baseball, Basketball and Football reflected traditional values: good conduct, cooperation, conformity, teamwork, character-building and sportsmanship. The new Extreme sports are rooted in a diametrically opposite set of values which include fierce individualism, alienation, defiance and some degree of inwardly-focused aggression. Unlike the Scooter craze, which has nothing to do with the changing social fabric, these new sports are an authentic slice of the wider youth culture, and not just a fad." On the other hand, the new youth culture is not synonymous with the larger youth demographic.

If Extreme sports are being propelled by new youth values, the traditional "blood" sports of Hunting, Shooting and Fishing reflect changing adult mores. These traditional pursuits, in Lauer's words, "are like a huge glacier, slowly being melted by the irreversible warming trend of humanistic evolution." In the past year, the trendiest of the Shooting sports (Sporting Clays) earned the dubious distinction of losing the most participants (-24%) while a close cousin (Trap/Skeet Shooting) fell by 19%, and Target Shooting declined by 11%. Hunting with a shotgun or rifle remained flat (-2%), but has fallen by 35% since 1987. During 1999-2000, the Bow Hunting population contracted by 11%. However, many of the shooting sports have relatively small sample bases, cautioned Lauer.

With 54.8 million adherents, Fishing remains the third most popular activity in the U.S., surpassed only by Recreational Walking and Swimming. In the past year, Fishing reflected zero-growth (-1%), and for the 1987-2000 period, a loss of 8%. However, due to a 15% increase in the U.S. population during that period, the actual incidence of Fishing has declined by over 20% -- a finding of high statistical significance.

Further analysis of the data indicates that after the elimination of Extreme and Snow Sports from the top 20 growth list, 6 of the remaining 10 activities are driven by an "older" constituency. Whereas the traditional Health Club member or home exerciser was once an 18-34 year-old "hardbody", today's fitness movement (and many other active pursuits) are underwritten by people over 35, and most strikingly, by those over 55. Between 1987-2000, the number of Health Club members aged 18-34 increased by only 12%; for people aged 55+, membership skyrocketed by 379%!

Elliptical Motion Trainers -- by far the hottest fitness equipment trend -- has surged to 6.2 million users in 2000, an increase of 22% from 1999 and 160% over 1997. This relatively new cardiovascular equipment involves an elliptical-shaped pedaling motion which has been described as a cross between a Nordic Ski Machine and Stair-Climber. This "no-impact" device is particularly friendly to older fitness enthusiasts -- particularly those with knee problems. Yoga, Aquatic Exercise and Treadmills are also kinder and gentler low-impact activities that credit recent growth to an influx of older converts. In the year 2000, two other populations with a high percentage of older participants -- Golf and R.V. Camping -- each increased by 8%.

But according to the Superstudy® of Sports Participation, mixed signals continue to emanate from the world of fitness. The three forms of outdoors exercise, Running (-1%) Fitness Walking (+1%) and Fitness Biking (-6%) have not advanced. Group Exercise -- a recent health club rage --

appears to have cooled, as Aerobics and Spinning declined by 8% and 22% respectively. After a fiery ascent to 7.6 million participants in 1999, Cardio Kickboxing has reached its apogee, leveling off to 7.2 million in 2000. Slower growth for this predominantly female activity was predicted by the 1999 ASD study, which revealed an average participation frequency of only 33 days -- not the hallmark of an enduring fitness trend.

Other fitness activities were in positive territory: Yoga/Tai Chi (+16%), Aquatics (+15%), Weight/Resistance Machines (+10%), and Treadmill Exercise (+9%). Free Weight Training edged up 4% for the year, but rose by 8% from 1998-2000. Within the Free Weights category, the use of light Hand Weights (fueled by women and older participants) increased by 5% for the year and 16% since 1998.

Overall, exactly 50 million Americans over the age of 6 participated at least 100 times in any single fitness activity, nearly identical to the 1999 measurement. But in opposition to the lackluster Megatrend, 32.8 million Health Club members were projected for the U.S. -- a 7% increase over the 1999 measurement of 30.6 million. More dramatically, the number of people who engaged the services of a Personal Trainer surged by 29%, to 5.3 million.

How then do we explain the paradox of both a booming Health Club industry and brisk Personal Trainer business in the face of a stalled fitness movement? Easily, says Lauer: "Health Clubs and Personal Trainers are benefiting from a failure of self-motivation among many fitness participants. It's difficult for people, on their own, to defy the Pleasure Principle -- to do something painful, inconvenient, time-consuming, or all three. People need external motivation, structure and reinforcement. Some also need social interaction."

The Superstudy® of Sports Participation was conducted in January 2001 and based on a nationally representative sample of 14,772 people over the age of 6, who were among 25,000 respondents targeted in a sample drawn from the consumer mail panel of NFO Research, Inc. 103 sports and activities were measured along over 20 demographic, attitudinal and behavioral dimensions. Data were also collected on health club membership and other subjects pertinent to physical fitness. This annual tracking study has been conducted by ASD every year since 1987, and sponsored by the Sporting Goods Manufacturers Association of North Palm Beach, Florida. For more information, log onto www.americansportsdata.com.

***

TRENDS IN U.S. SPORTS/FITNESS PARTICIPATION 1999 - 2000
LARGEST GAINS

	Participants* (000)	1-Year Change 1999-2000 (%)
1. Snowboarding	7,151	+51.2
2. Skateboarding	11,649	+49.2
3. Wakeboarding	3,581	+32.3
4. Snowmobiling	7,032	+28.1
5. Gymnastics	6,689	+27.3
6. Artificial Wall Climbing	6,117	+27.0
7. Surfing	2,180	+25.6
8. Elliptical Motion Trainers	6,176	+21.6
9. Softball (Fast-Pitch)	3,795	+18.1
10. Snowshoeing	1,970	+17.8
11. Skiing (Cross-Country)	4,613	+15.7
12. Yoga/Tai Chi	7,400	+15.6
13. Football (Tackle)	5,673	+15.0
14. Paintball	7,121	+11.9
15. Weight/Resistance Machines	25,182	+ 9.7
16. Treadmill Exercise	40,816	+ 9.0
17. Camping (R.V.)	19,035	+ 8.3
18. Golf	30,365	+ 7.6
19. Fishing (Fly)	6,581	+ 7.3[†]
20. Skiing (Downhill)	14,749	+ 6.4[†]

* At least once in year 2000
[†] Change not statistically significant at 95% Confidence Level

LARGEST DECLINES

	Participants* (000)	1-Year Change 1999-2000 (%)
1. Shooting (Sporting Clays)	2,843	-24.2
2. Stationary Cycling (Spinning)	5,431	-21.8
3. Shooting (Trap/Skeet)	3,827	-19.3
4. Trail Running	5,232	-16.1
5. Aerobics (Low-Impact)	9,752	-15.8
6. Target Shooing (Pistol)	10,433	-13.6
7. Archery	6,047	-12.8
8. Roller Skating (2x2 Wheels)	10,834	-12.7
9. Hunting (Bow)	4,120	-11.0[†]
10. Aerobics (High-Impact)	5,581	-10.7[†]
11. Baseball	10,881	-9.8
12. Racquetball	5,155	-8.5[†]
13. Volleyball (Beach)	8,763	-8.0[†]

* At least once in year 2000
[†] Change not statistically significant at 95% Confidence Level

CHAPTER 20

CURRENT ISSUES IN YOUTH SPORTS

Character Development vs. Physiological Benefits: The Need for Balanced Emphasis

To the limited extent that sports are acknowledged to have intrinsic developmental value, we hear the familiar (if not yet understood) character building tenet: sports can provide a venue for social adjustment, character building, a sense of belonging, usefulness, psychological well-being, and ultimately a springboard to the highest values of citizenship.

But we never hear much about the <u>physiological</u> benefits of sports/exercise; these incentives are either understated or absent. Perhaps the causal connection between sports participation and health is taken for granted, or maybe the opposite condition exists: a lack of conviction that sports programs are physically demanding enough to make a difference.

It has been pointed out that in a nation of children preoccupied by sports and sports heroes, too few participate in sports. The fact is that overall, youth sports participation is in severe decline. While reasons are too complex to be addressed here, the important point is that this downtrend parallels both an alarming demise of phys ed programs in our schools <u>and</u> a child obesity crisis.

Not long after its creation over a century ago, physical education was abdicated by policymakers, legislators, healthcare providers and the philanthropic community to the public schools, which by the end of the 20th century -- had begun to fail abysmally in this obligation. A partial result of this failure is the declining level of youthful physical activity, and a concomitant child obesity crisis that according to some criteria, has achieved epidemic proportions. Nationwide, only about 1 out of 4 teenagers take part in some form of physical education; from 1980 - 1999, the percentage of adolescents who were overweight nearly tripled (from 5% to 14%).

According to the Centers for Disease Control, daily participation in High School physical education classes dropped from 42% in 1991 to 27% in 1997. In a parallel finding, American Sports Data, Inc. reported that in 1987, 23.3% of all children aged 12-17 participated in a fitness activity on at least 100 occasions; by 1997, the figure had dropped to 19.2%. Not only does this de-emphasis of physical education in our schools contribute to what is now publicly characterized as an epidemic of child obesity; vanishing phys ed programs only blunt an already flagging enthusiasm for school sports. Meager, discretionary school budgets -- originally intended for athletics or other extracurricular activities -- are being diverted for academic use.

To address the crisis of declining physical activity among the nation's youth, two major initiatives are in progress. The PE4LIFE campaign, instituted by leaders in the sporting goods industry and the Sporting Goods Manufacturers Association, played a significant role in the recent passage of the Physical Education For Progress Act (PEP). The legislation allocates $50 million a year to local school districts across the U.S. that initiate and improve PE programs for K-12 students.

In addition, the CDC has recently announced a $125 million Youth Media Campaign to promote physical activity and nutrition among the nation's 9-13 year-olds.

With these exceptions, youth development is framed almost exclusively in psychosocial outcomes; physiological payoffs are rarely even acknowledged. Should a greater emphasis be placed on the health and fitness benefits of sports, the latter could more easily connect with youth development.

A Dearth of Qualified Coaches
Many youth sports programs never see the light of day for lack of volunteers. A good number fail because of poorly qualified coaches, or an over-reliance on untrained volunteers. As many as 90% of the nation's 2.5 million volunteer coaches lack formal preparation, according to a study by Ewing, Seefeldt and Brown. With the exception of the National Alliance for Youth Sports, no certification or accreditation agencies exist for this purpose; or at least none have been unearthed by this preliminary research. Even worse, there is also the oxymoron of an acute shortage of unqualified coaches -- people simply don't volunteer. The National Youth Sports Safety Foundation estimates that 3-5 million children suffer sports-related injuries each year, many serious enough to require emergency room treatment. Undoubtedly, many of these injuries are preventable; we can only speculate that a fair number are related to the quality of coaching. The upcoming ASD study on sports injuries will greatly illuminate this general area.

A Shifting Landscape: From Traditional to "Extreme" Sports

The last decade of the 20th century has witnessed vast changes in American values and the popular culture. As part of a larger social and technological transformation, the thinking, lifestyles, and leisure behavior of children have been profoundly affected. And perhaps, as some would argue, the changes in youthful psychology and behavior are transforming the larger society. Whatever the sociological reality, the landscape of youth sports participation is being altered dramatically.

In the new millennium, Baseball, Basketball and Football are still among the most popular participatory sports; but the number of people who participate in these activities is plummeting. In the year 2000, there were 11 million Baseball players in the U.S., 28% fewer than in 1987. Though still a major force, the army of 19.7 million Softball players has dwindled from 31 million in 1987 -- a fall of 36%. Volleyball participation is also down by 36% between 1987 - 2000, and during the same period, the pastime of Touch Football declined by 24%. It must be emphasized that much of this decline stems from a drop-off in casual, pickup play. Organized participation is declining less precipitously, while several team sports -- notably Soccer and Lacrosse -- have grown.

Traditional team sports such as Baseball, Basketball and Football reflect traditional values: cooperation, teamwork, character-building, and healthy competition. Unlike traditional sports, the new genre of so-called "Extreme" sports (i.e. In-Line Skating, Skateboarding, BMX, Snowboarding, Paintball, Wakeboarding) is rooted in a diametrically opposite set of values. The common defining feature of these alternative sports is the "adrenaline rush" produced by the thrill and excitement of being "on the edge" -- a reflection (if we accept the pop cultural profile) of the new "in-your-face" ethic characterized by fierce individualism, alienation, defiance and inwardly-focused aggressive behavior.

According to the SUPERSTUDY® of Sports Participation by American Sports Data, Inc. Snowboarding (+51%), Skateboarding (+49%) and Wakeboarding (+32%) -- three of the so-called extreme or Millennial sports -- were the fastest growing in the U.S. during the first year of the New Millennium. "Extreme," "Millennial" or "Action" sports appear to be an authentic slice of the wider youth culture -- the athletic complement of other irreverent elements of attitude, dress, music, humor and general lifestyle that are emblematic of Generation "Y." It should be remembered however, that the amorphous and largely undocumented Generation "Y" psychographic is only a fraction of the youth population.

That said, Extreme sports cannot be considered a "fad"; but whether or not this statement will make a lasting imprint (as did many aspects of the 1960's counterculture) remains to be seen. In any event, we may be witnessing a seismic shift in sports participation patterns, with enormous implications for the content of youth development sports programs, not to mention the direction of sporting goods product markets.

Quite paradoxically, the argument is heard that many youngsters are defecting to these activities for peace and solitude -- to escape not only supervision and authority, but the unbearable pressures inflicted by parents and coaches in traditional team sports.

A Shortage of Athletic Facilities

Paralleling -- or perhaps contributing to -- the decline of school sports is an apparent crisis in the availability and condition of athletic fields and facilities. As a corollary to the twin neglect by public school systems of physical education and sports programs, many facilities -- particularly in urban areas -- are said to be dilapidated and overgrown, some having languished and deteriorated into parking lots. A recent New York City investigation for example, revealed that 54 of the city's 59 high school ball fields are in severe disrepair.

While traditional team sports have lost participants, many dropouts have been pickup players; revealing (with the exception of Baseball) a fairly stable core of organized players. At the same time, the growth of other activities (particularly Soccer, but also Lacrosse, Cheerleading, Golf, and Fast-Pitch Softball) has been amplified by increases in female participation, and collectively, exert intense pressure on existing athletic facilities. In addition, whereas 15 years ago, sports leagues for children under 10 were rare, today, kindergartners routinely play T-Ball and Soccer -- on a field. Finally, the new Extreme Sports are mandating non-traditional venues such as Skate parks and Paintball fields.

An overloaded or decaying infrastructure will ultimately strangle youth sports participation. Team rosters are being downsized, the formation of new teams prevented, existing participation undermined by the sheer inconvenience and difficulty associated with unreasonable scheduling, insufficient open spaces and facilities.

Current Issues in Youth Sports

A badly needed legislative elixir for this problem has recently come from the House passage of the CARA bill (Conservation and Reinvestment Act) that would provide an annual outlay of $2.8 Billion to acquire and protect open space, construct playing fields and revitalize urban parks.

The Gender-Equity Issue

Statistics from the National Federation of State High School Associations reflect massive increases in female participation for various interscholastic sports over the past two decades -- unquestionably the result of wider opportunities for girls engendered by the passage of Title IX (of the Federal Education Amendments of 1972), which provided that "no person in the United States shall, on the basis of sex, be excluded from participation in, be denied the benefits of, or be subjected to discrimination under, any education program or activity receiving federal financial assistance".

Still, male participation in youth sports is by far predominant -- a disparity that persists for a complex variety of cultural, physiological and psychological reasons. On the "supply" side, the failure of institutions to fully redress the inequity of opportunity for young women bears only partial responsibility for the continuing gender gap. On the "demand" side, subtle issues of female identity, self-esteem, social awareness and consciousness-raising form a less visible wedge between ideal and reality.

Nonetheless, the progress made by young women in sports is unmistakable. According to the National Federation of State High School Associations, young women comprised 42% of all high school athletes in 2000-2001, leaping from only 7% in the pre-Title IX era (1971). In absolute terms, the number of female athletes skyrocketed by 847% during this period. The American Sports Data, Inc. Sector Analysis Report reflected that of the 25 million frequent team sports participants in the year 2000, 43% were female. However, this percentage declined to 40% in 2001, and slipped to 36% in 2002.

But Title IX is not immune to criticism. Indeed, while moderate opponents view the legislation as a good idea gone awry, more vocal critics -- prominently represented by the male-dominated Wrestling community -- see Title IX as a once-righteous ideal allowed to mutate toward the lunatic extreme.

The most commonly used Title IX remedy compels universities that accept federal support to maintain proportionality between athletic team rosters and the male-female ratios of student bodies, and the practice has resulted -- according to the opposition -- in both gross injustices to very talented male athletes, and conversely, outlandish efforts to recruit barely-interested females. Detractors of Title IX are fond of citing the effort of a desert-bound Arizona college to form (i.e. recruit from scratch) a women's Rowing team! In a less jocular vein, they claim that many talented male athletes -- particularly smaller men relegated to Wrestling, Gymnastics or Swimming -- are totally deprived of sports participation opportunities, because in pursuit of gender-parity, schools have eliminated many of these "secondary" teams.

Defenders of Title IX contend that the issue is <u>money</u>; that to redress male-female imbalances, meaningful cuts could be made from bloated male rosters in football and basketball...but feckless administrators dare not trifle with these huge, sacred cash cows.

The courts, while expressing a modicum of sympathy for the male position, have found in favor of Title IX. Its abolition, or even significant alteration, would not -- it has been decreed -- constitute a significant practical remedy for the plaintiffs. Policy-makers in the Bush administration have recently upheld this view.

The Inner-City: Unequal Access to Athletic Facilities

Historically, Inner-City youth sports programs have been inhibited by numerous factors. First and foremost, the dominant presence of large youth organizations such as Little League, AYSO and Pop Warner has perpetuated the widespread (middle-class) belief that youth sports opportunities are abundant, and need not be supplemented with additional (inner-city/lower-income) programs.

Naturally, many private fee-based youth sports opportunities are beyond the reach of low-income youth, and must be augmented in low-income areas by youth service organizations, municipal facilities, neighborhood recreation centers, and of course, informal pickup play.

An important objective of sports research should be to quantify and document the extent to which minority youth rely on not-for-profit athletic facilities and pickup play, vis-à-vis their more affluent counterparts. Indeed, a comparison of public school-based sports participation between high and low-income neighborhoods should prove equally informative.

An even more compelling hypothesis for research deals with the particularly acute lack of athletic opportunity for African-American and Latino women in low-income communities, impeded by the dual barrier of race and gender.

* * *

CHAPTER 21

SPORTS PARTICIPATION: THE METAPHOR OF YOUTH DEVELOPMENT

It has been observed that after religion, sport is the most powerful cultural force in American society. This sweeping generalization covers two domains: sports spectatorship or viewership, and sports participation. The latter phenomenon is arguably more important, because it lends itself to that ineffable process called "youth development". From an adult viewpoint, youth sports participation serves four broad purposes:

- It provides children with "fun" and instant gratification;
- It fulfills what social psychologists call the "affiliative" need -- friendship, and a sense of belonging;
- It offers the near-term prospect of healthier minds and bodies through physical exercise;
- For the longer term, its cumulative benefits hold the promise of achieving the favorable "outcomes" associated with youth development.

Aside from the issues of overzealous parents and untutored coaches, most people have no trouble with the first proposition. That sport is fun is almost a banal observation -- requiring little in the way of social commentary. Academically, the simple joy of sports can suffer profound psychological erudition -- or it can be expressed far more powerfully in the eloquence of a simple anecdote:

> *"I knew that sports were very important, even though I also knew when I was six that I wanted to be a doctor. So I worked hard in school. But nothing was like that moment on the basketball court*

when you drove to the hoop. There was nothing like that in anything else I ever did. So I knew the value, the importance of athletics."

These are the words of Dr. James P. Comer, Professor of Child Psychiatry at Yale University, describing his Indiana boyhood, where he played Basketball under street lights. Generally, a quote from such an eminent educator would be reserved for a more penetrating discussion of youth development, not squandered on so obvious a notion.

There may already be a vague quaintness about Comer's anecdote for many of today's youth, as "the thrill of driving to the hoop" is being superceded by the adrenaline rush of BMX, Snowboarding, Paintball and the other new, so-called "Extreme Sports". But the enjoyment of sport is timeless, and its potential as a youth development medium, vast.

Youth development is implicit in all organized sports participation. While much of this discussion concerns more conscious and deliberate applications of sports as "interventions" for troubled youths and those headed for trouble, the concept is equally viable for "positive" youth development in conventional school settings, sports leagues, and organized play generally.

The enormous power of sports can serve not only as a magnet for youth recruitment; if properly harnessed, it offers remarkable leverage for remedial youth development outcomes in sports-dedicated programs. In a word: because of their passion for sports, kids will stick with and thrive in an enrichment program, if that's what it takes to stay on the team. And if we can make sports relevant to the particular educational or enrichment curricula that underlie what is known as "positive" youth development, the probability of successful outcomes will be multiplied proportionately.

That sports fill a basic social need is also obvious, but not widely discussed. Indeed, the major incentive for many children who participate in team sports -- especially those who are lacking in athletic skills, and also perhaps in self-esteem -- has little to do with athletics, and everything to do with a newly acquired network of social relationships.

The third premise, that physical activity is a source of improved health and well-being -- while also accepted -- does not quite achieve the unanimity of the first two concepts. Simply stated, all sports are not created equal: some are insufficiently demanding to exact even the minimum fitness benefit, while at the other extreme, certain sports pose the threat of injury. Both issues have kindled narrow academic debates.

In any event, long ago, even before the advent of modern conveniences and the mass production of the automobile, it was observed that despite the natural appeal, innate moral, physical and spiritual benefits of sports participation, children -- when left to their own devices, or the influence of peer groups, family or other institutions -- did not get enough exercise. This belief was implicit in the very creation of physical education -- early on abdicated by policymakers, legislators, healthcare providers and the philanthropic community to the public schools -- which by the end of the 20th century had begun to fail abysmally in this obligation. A partial result of this failure is the declining level of youthful physical activity, and a concomitant child obesity crisis that according to some criteria, has achieved epidemic proportions. Nationwide, only about 1 out of 4 teenagers take part in some form of physical education. From 1980 - 1999, the percentage of adolescents who were overweight nearly tripled (from 5% to 14%).

The fourth idea -- sports-as-medium-for-youth-development -- is far more complex. Long ago, it was said that the battles of the British Empire (most notably Waterloo) were won many years earlier on the playing fields of Eton. Two centuries later, the metaphor persists: early experiences of American children on the Baseball diamond, Basketball court and Soccer field will mold good citizens, productive, well-adjusted members of society. In theory, (and with some empirical foundation) youth sports promote self-esteem and self-confidence, build character, engender responsible social behavior, inspire the living habits, social values, civic participation, healthy and wholesome lifestyles that culminate in the better life, and if we're lucky -- a few outstanding leaders. But this compelling thesis has never been definitively proved.

Within the constellation of <u>remedial</u> youth development, sports are barely visible -- dwarfed by much larger influences and institutions including: family, peer groups, public schools, healthcare systems, and community organizations. In the wider "problem-focused" world of youth development, the list includes counseling and treatment in the areas of drug addiction, alcohol abuse, violence, gang membership, teen pregnancy, academic failure, homelessness and joblessness, to name just a few.

Sports Participation: The Metaphor of Youth Development

Against such an array of grave subjects and solemn mandates, sports participation can only seem frivolous; and this begins to explain why -- in the overall context of therapeutic youth development thinking and funding -- sports programs are given short shrift, or avoided altogether. But this is not the only reason.

As a cultural concept, "sport" is synonymous with "fun", "leisure", "recreation" and "play" -- distinctly separated from the more serious work of society. The immense popularity of spectator sports in the U.S. tends to widen this gulf in the public mind, with tarnished images of sports celebrities and professional teams further undermining the value of sports as a legitimate youth development vehicle.

Sports participation is linked to youth development only as a metaphor -- and this is essentially why it is not taken seriously by the professional/philanthropic community, and a major reason for the scarcity of "pure" stand-alone youth development programs that highlight a sports theme (i.e. Harlem RBI, Think Detroit, Students Run LA, etc.). Because a metaphor by definition is not obligated to explain precisely how, for example, the captaincy of a Basketball team translates to leadership in the boardroom, the links between sports participation and character education (i.e. respect, discipline, compassion, perseverance, decision-making, problem-solving, etc.) remain vague abstractions.

Nonetheless, if we think about how sports can interact with educational or enrichment programs, a four-level hierarchy is suggested:

LEVEL I
> Stand-alone youth sports programs that are purely recreational and performance-based -- unassociated with any formal youth development agenda;

LEVEL II
> Sports participation deployed as a "hook" to attract youth at drop-in centers, after-school activities or other enrichment programs;

LEVEL III
> Sport is the centerpiece of a youth development program, but remains disconnected from the developmental or educational component, functioning merely as a lever to encourage program attendance/performance; the character education aspect is indirect, nominal, or insufficiently pursued.

LEVEL IV
> Sports become directly relevant to youth development. Elements of the sports experience are synthesized with character education, skills acquisition, academic subjects or other enrichment themes. (Baseball statistics are used to teach math skills; a Scuba Diving course incorporates the rudiments of marine biology/oceanography, etc.).

Much of youth sports participation defies easy classification; and even if definitive pigeon-holing were possible, the hierarchical structure does not imply a ranking of program superiority.

Level I programs are the most numerous; they include school sports and organized participation such as AYSO, Little League and POP Warner, but in most instances lack a formal component of youth development or character education.

Sports Participation: The Metaphor of Youth Development

Level II programs are typified by the Bird Street Youth Center in Boston, L.A.'s Best, the Youth Sports Connection in San Francisco, Athletes Against Drugs (Chicago) and countless neighborhood youth centers.

Level III programs include Sports4Kids in Oakland, Harlem RBI in New York, Courageous Sailing Center of Boston, Kids In Sports (L.A.), Metro Lacrosse (Boston), Think Detroit, Ice Hockey in Harlem, Row As One Institute, (Mass.), and the Native American Sports Council. Qualifiers in this category are scarce, probably numbering fewer than 100 nationwide. Distinctions between Levels II & III are blurred, and the latter could include Boys & Girls Clubs, the CYO, PAL, etc.

Level IV initiatives are exceedingly rare, likely enumerated with a single digit.

As a corollary, "best practices" for sports participation and youth development are unique, because these two parallel lines almost never meet. In fact, due to negative publicity, many Level I programs (Baseball, Soccer and Hockey, for example) appear counterproductive, even antithetical to character-building.

In most remedial youth development settings, sports participation is a peripheral adjunct -- at best, an essential lure for attracting kids to a community center or program; at worst, tolerated as an annoying distraction from the "real" priorities of youth development: education, jobs, pregnancy, drugs, violence, etc. Even in the rare dedicated, sport-centered program focusing on character-education, the sports team or league is conceptually detached from the particular prevention, intervention or enrichment theme(s). Potentially, Level IV programs (if they existed in either remedial or conventional sports environments) would define the best practices.

Linking the playing fields of Eton to the battles of the British Empire is probably more analogy than metaphor; the latter day connection between the sports participation of underprivileged children and the goals of youth development is far more abstruse. How exactly can we link Soccer with "character-building"? Golf, Tennis or Lacrosse with benevolence, fair-play, civic participation, or integrity?

Little contemporary research exists on the practical application of the sports metaphor. On the adult level, Dr. Robert Keidel's Game Plan: Sports Strategies for Business (1985), related the dynamics of sports teams to management styles and organizational forms. Character Development and Physical Activity (Shields & Bredemeir -- 1995) offers the most exhaustive academic treatment of the application of sport to moral development and character education. Ewing (1997) has discussed the role of sports in social and moral development, emphasizing the on-field contributions of parents and coaches to the younger child's evolving self-esteem, social competence, sense of fairness, honesty and other values.

Because abstract thinking is less developed in very young children, they cannot and perhaps should not be "taught" precisely how sports experiences translate to the building blocks of character development; suffice it that they internalize these values

Sports Participation: The Metaphor of Youth Development

through feedback, coaching, emulation, or other natural processes. In addition to the acquisition of self-confidence and self-esteem, the moral principles inherent in sharing, abiding by rules, "right-and-wrong", consequences of behavior, cooperation, honesty, respect, and fairness can be learned on the playing field. Later, the lessons can be taught more formally.

If we borrow a pedagogical technique pioneered by the great academic philosopher John Dewey, sports can be made relevant to academic subjects, life skills instruction, and to varying degrees -- most aspects of youth development. Dewey's method was simple, but required significant creativity -- thus explaining why it never reached the educational mainstream. His purpose was to erase the distinction between the natural condition of the "real world", the artificial, coercive -- and to children, seemingly oppressive -- nature of the classroom. He enlivened and enriched the educational experience by taking mundane pursuits and occupations such as cooking, carpentry, sewing and weaving, making them <u>relevant</u> to academic subjects such as arithmetic, physics, chemistry and biology. Cooking for example, might invoke arithmetic (measuring and weighing ingredients) or physics (temperatures of boiling water); carpentry the subject of geometry; weaving and sewing, geography, etc.

A curriculum linking the various sports to academic subjects would not be a great departure from the original Dewey model. One such application -- created by a veteran of the Harlem RBI program -- uses Baseball statistics to teach math skills. Another New York program, Urban Dove, applies a similar technique: marine biology and oceanography are seamlessly interwoven in a program that trains and then certifies children in Scuba Diving. Students Run Los Angeles is unique in that it helps children build self-esteem by training for and completing a full 26.2 mile Marathon, where elements of the sports experience and desired outcomes are one and the same, unseparated by conceptual leaps or metaphors. These are rare Level IV phenomena.

A leap from sports to leadership, career goals, or morality is a bit more difficult, but not beyond the imagination of a good theorist. And there is nothing, we have been told, so practical as a good theory -- even during the twilight of progressive education.

An anecdote borrowed from the outstanding contribution of Milbrey W. McLaughlin (<u>Community Counts</u>) illustrates how the sports experience can be linked to the goals/outcomes of youth development. Successful programs, implied the research, are accompanied by an interplay of specific rules and strict expectations. The following example of a Basketball program is taken from a case study:

"If a player stops going to school, he cannot play. Missing two practices means the bench for the next game. Not showing up in uniform means the bench plus push-ups. Youth were adamant about having and enforcing such rules. For example, a basketball coach had a lot of explaining to do when he called a benched player into the game against a tough opponent. The coach reasoned, wrongly, that the team would consider winning the game more important than sticking to the rules. As they told him in angry recriminations after the game 'rules are rules' and even if it meant a loss, they should be applied consistently."

Sports Participation: The Metaphor of Youth Development

But will the children who so fiercely defended the "rules" understand that in the larger context of society, the "rules" are the legal system? If so, can they -- without any prompting or guidance -- make the conceptual leap from the Basketball court to the judicial system? Will they understand that, to make the larger system work, the same underlying moral principle is required? The answer is that we probably cannot rely on the vagaries of osmosis and unstructured learning to ensure that an adolescent makes this abstract connection.

This vignette provides the ingredients for a participant module, coaching seminar or parental workshop that addresses rules, fairness, integrity, the judicial system or similar topics relevant to the goals of youth development. There are countless others to be gleaned from the annals of everyday sports experience -- certainly enough to build a curriculum from the century-old experimental philosophy of John Dewey.

Fortunately, a quantum leap in this direction has already been made by Dr. Jeffrey P. Beedy, who reminds us that, in contemporary education, sports and physical education are classified as "extracurricular" -- disembodied from the "true" academic curriculum, without even the faintest recognition that sports have didactic value for general education.

In 1995, Beedy pioneered a Boston After School program called Sports PLUS. This unique integration of sports participation and classroom learning creates a "unit" for each of five character themes: teamwork, respect, responsibility, fair play and perseverance, where children explore such complex issues as discrimination, justice and violence. Reading serves as the primary instructional vehicle -- honing language skills, improving thinking ability, and teaching interpersonal values. In addition to sports participation, other teaching media are sports vignettes, sports dilemmas, workbooks, journal writing, sports cartoons, current sports-related events, and role playing.

The early results of this 24-student pilot were very encouraging. Participants increased their amount of reading, demonstrated an increased understanding of character themes, and improved their ability to work together in small teams.

To bridge sports participation and youth development we need only refine this prototype, tweak it for slightly older children, adapt it to a neighborhood setting, then the crescendo: a Level IV model for national replication.

* * *

CHAPTER 22

"GENERATION Y" DRIVES INCREASINGLY POPULAR "EXTREME" SPORTS

FOR IMMEDIATE RELEASE   August 1, 2002

* * *

<u>GROWTH OF NEW "MILLENNIAL" PURSUITS OUTPACES TRADITIONAL ACTIVITIES</u>

* * *

<u>But Team Sports Still Attract the Most Kids</u>

HARTSDALE, N.Y. -- Sports and leisure preferences mirror an evolving society, reflecting not only explosive changes in the youth culture, but also the basic need for novelty and change. From 1998 - 2001, the largest gains in sports participation have come from the new "Extreme" Sports, (variously dubbed "Millennial", "Alternative", "New Age", and "Action" Sports): Skateboarding (+73%), Artificial Wall Climbing (+57%), Wakeboarding (+38%), Paintball (+30%) and Snowboarding (+25%). These were among the findings of the 15th annual SUPERSTUDY® of Sports Participation, conducted in January 2002, among 14,276 Americans nationwide, by American Sports Data, Inc. (ASD).

That the new Action Sports have gained ground during the same period at the expense of traditional American pastimes such as Baseball (-7%), Basketball (-9%) or Touch Football (-4%) is undeniable; but in the aggregate, team sports (which happen to include the trendier activities of Soccer, Lacrosse and Fast-Pitch Softball) continue to enlist the highest number of followers. In 2001, <u>frequent</u> participants in team sports (generally defined as having played 25+ days per year) totaled 26.5 million -- still outnumbering the fast-growing army of Extreme Sports recruits, which including In-Line Skaters (a population of dubious "Extreme" characteristics), mustered only 14.2 million frequent participants.

Still, the Extreme Sports juggernaut seems unstoppable. As members of the Old Guard peer through their field glasses, they wonder not if -- but exactly <u>when</u> they will be overrun, and who the invaders are. But when they slide the template of cultural values over the map of Extreme Sports, their most alarming intelligence reports are confirmed: these hordes are the dreaded legions of "Generation Y" -- a growing army of 70 million destined to become the most formidable demographic in American history. Also known as the "New Millennials", "Generation Next", the "Digital Generation" or the "Echo Boom", these future rulers of the 21st century are -- depending on the source -- between 6-17, 8-20, or even 6-24 years of age.

According to pop culture, the defining feature of "Generation Y" is a disdain for authority, while the second most distinctive strand in the Millennial personality -- and the one most relevant to sports participation -- is a propensity for risk-taking. The common denominator of all Extreme Sports is the thrill-seeking experience, culminating in the adrenaline-rush.

These sports may in fact, be organized on a continuum -- not according to degree of danger, injury potential or recklessness, but based on levels of adrenaline production. In the hierarchy, the most _extreme_ sports are probably Sky-Diving and Bungee-Jumping while Snowboarding and BMX fall toward the middle; In-Line Skating, the category progenitor, would be positioned at the "tame" end of the spectrum. Paintball, neither a board sport nor one featuring gravity-induced adrenaline, offers not only Millennial panache, but a unique channel for the sublimation of "Y's" allegedly aggressive instincts -- emerging as perhaps the quintessential sport of "Generation Y".

Most Extreme Sports are solitary activities that not only allow the participant to avoid social interaction, but provide an escape from supervision and authority. This is in stark contrast to the broad (but vaguely credible) generalization that years ago, traditional American pastimes were symbols of teamwork, cooperation, respect, authority and wholesome living; team sports were in essence, the metaphor of positive youth development. These were "Silent Generation" values of the strait-laced, button-downed Beaver family, and also much later of the Brady Bunch, icon of the "Boomers" which -- despite a hint of evolving sassiness -- still bore the authoritarian imprint.

By the time of the "Simpsons" and "Generation X", authority started to unravel. Decorum began to slip away from the Little League baseball field; shrill, whiny tennis players were no longer suitable role models, and a wave of barbarism -- epitomized by the shattering glass of a slam-dunked backboard -- swept over professional team sports. In some cities, Major League outfielders were in constant peril of being shelled by their own fans. And in grotesque contrast to an unbroken phalanx of coats and ties in stadium photographs of the 1940's and 1950's, the New Millennium portrait offers only a grandstand spectacle of the half-naked, half-painted bellowing role models of "Generation Y".

If "Generation X" represented a radical, postmodern break with tradition, "Generation Y" -- raised on "Barney", hooked on "Real World" and Professional Wrestling -- is easily postapocalyptic. However sound the typology, Extreme Sports seem to match the Millennial profile. They bear a distinctive "in-your-face" cachet, as sports participation -- in and of itself -- becomes a celebration of defiance and unconventional behavior, a <u>statement</u> that announces: "I'm doing this because it's cool and different, to thumb my nose at the world, and for the absolute thrill and excitement of it -- even if it means putting myself at risk." To the extent that Gen Y represents the larger youth cohort, this is an important piece of social analysis.

There is almost no question that to one degree or another, the new Alternative Sports are an authentic slice of the wider youth culture, and not just a fad. Whether or not they -- like the radical values changes of the 1960's counterculture -- will be an enduring legacy in the larger society is the key question. "Whether or not we buy into the pop sociology" says ASD president Harvey Lauer, "we better pay attention to this group, because Millennials are the biggest thing since their parents, the Boomers." Indeed, Millennials number around 70 million, and are much larger than "Generation "X". At its peak, "Y" will surpass Baby Boomers in absolute numbers. Most important, between now and 2010, this group will grow at twice the rate of the general population -- and in addition to defining the 21st century, these future leaders currently participate in Extreme Sports.

The Superstudy® of Sports Participation was conducted in January 2002 and based on a nationally representative sample of 14,276 people over the age of 6, who were among 25,000 respondents targeted in a sample drawn from the consumer mail panel of NFO Research, Inc. 103 sports and activities were measured along over 20 demographic, attitudinal and behavioral dimensions. Data were also collected on health club membership and other subjects pertinent to physical fitness. This annual tracking study has been conducted by ASD every year since 1987, and sponsored by the Sporting Goods Manufacturers Association of North Palm Beach, Florida. For more information, log onto www.americansportsdata.com.

* * *

SELECTED "ALTERNATIVE" SPORTS
(Participated at least once in last 12 months)
(000)

	1987	1990	1993	1998	2001	3-Year Change	14-Year Change
Skateboarding	10,888	9,267	5,388	7,190	12,459	+73%	+14%
Artificial Wall Climbing	n.a.	n.a.	n.a.	4,696	7,377	+57%	n.a.
Wakeboarding	n.a.	n.a.	n.a.	2,253	3,097	+38%	n.a.
Paintball	n.a.	n.a.	n.a.	5,923	7,678	+30%	n.a.
Snowboarding	n.a.	2,116	2,567	5,461	6,797	+25%	+221%[1]
Snowshoeing	n.a.	n.a.	n.a.	1,721	2,042	+19%[†]	n.a.
Mountain/Rock Climbing	n.a.	n.a.	n.a.	2,004	1,819	-9%[†]	n.a.
Roller Skating(In-Line)	n.a.	4,695	13,689	32,010	26,022	-19%	+454%[1]
Mountain Biking	1,512	4,146	7,408	8,611	6,189	-28%	+309%
Bicycling (BMX)	n.a.	n.a.	n.a.	n.a.	3,668	n.a.	n.a.
Surfing	1,459	1,224	n.a.	1,395	1,601	+15%[†]	+10%[†]

[1] 11-Year Change   [†] Not Statistically Significant

Source: American Sports Data, Inc. ~ SUPERSTUDY® of Sports Participation

Extreme vs. Traditional Sports

SELECTED "TRADITIONAL" SPORTS/ACTIVITIES
(Participated at least once in last 12 months)
(000)

	1987	1990	1993	1998	2001	3-Year Change	14-Year Change
Team							
Softball (Fast-Pitch)	n.a.	n.a.	n.a.	3,702	4,117	+11%	n.a.
Soccer	15,388	15,945	16,365	18,176	19,042	+5%	+24%
Football (Touch)	20,292	20,894	21,241	17,382	16,675	-4%	-18%
Softball (Total)	30,995	32,479	30,135	21,352	20,123	-6%	-35%
Baseball	15,098	15,454	15,586	12,318	11,405	-7%	-25%
Basketball	35,737	39,808	42,138	42,417	38,663	-9%	+8%
Volleyball (Total)	35,984	39,633	37,757	26,637	24,123	-9%	-33%
Racquet							
Racquetball	10,395	9,213	7,412	5,853	5,296	-9%	-49%
Tennis	21,147	21,742	19,346	16,937	15,098	-11%	-29%
Badminton	14,793	13,559	11,908	9,936	7,684	-23%	-48%
Indoors							
Bowling	47,823	53,537	49,022	50,593	55,452	+10%	+16%
Billiards/Pool	35,297	38,862	40,254	39,654	39,263	-1%	+11%
Table Tennis	n.a.	20,089	17,689	14,999	13,239	-12%	-34%[1]
Outdoors							
Kayaking	n.a.	n.a.	n.a.	3,501	4,727	+35%	n.a.
Trail Running	n.a.	n.a.	n.a.	5,249	5,773	+10%	n.a.
Camping (R.V.)	22,655	20,764	22,187	18,188	19,117	+5%	-16%
Walking (Recreational)	n.a.	n.a.	n.a.	80,864	84,182	+4%	n.a.
Camping (Tent)	35,232	36,915	34,772	42,677	43,472	+2%	+23%

[1] 11-Year Change

Source: American Sports Data, Inc. -- SUPERSTUDY® of Sports Participation

SELECTED "TRADITIONAL" SPORTS/ACTIVITIES (continued)
(Participated at least once in last 12 months)
(000)

	1987	1990	1993	1998	2001	3-Year Change	14-Year Change
Outdoors (cont.)							
Swimming (Recreational)	n.a.	n.a.	n.a.	94,371	93,571	-1%	n.a.
Bicycling (Recreational)	n.a.	n.a.	n.a.	54,575	52,948	-3%	n.a.
Hiking	n.a.	n.a.	n.a.	40,117	37,999	-5%	n.a.
Canoeing	n.a.	n.a.	n.a.	13,615	12,044	-12%	n.a.
Rafting	n.a.	n.a.	n.a.	5,570	4,580	-18%	n.a.
Water Skiing	19,902	19,314	16,626	10,161	8,301	-18%	-58%
Hunting/Fishing							
Hunting	25,241	23,220	23,189	16,681	16,672	0	-34%
Target Shooting	18,947	21,840	23,498	18,330	17,838	-3%	-6%
Fishing (Total)	58,402	58,816	55,442	55,488	53,137	-4%	-9%
Fly Fishing	11,359	8,039	6,598	7,269	5,999	-17%	-47%
Winter							
Skiing (Downhill)	17,676	18,209	17,567	14,836	13,202	-11%	-25%
Ice Skating	n.a.	n.a.	n.a.	18,710	16,573	-11%	n.a.
Skiing (Cross-Country)	8,344	7,292	6,489	4,728	4,123	-13%	-51%
Other							
Golf	26,261	28,945	28,610	29,961	29,382	-2%	+12%
Roller Skating (2x2 Wheels)	n.a.	27,101	24,223	14,752	11,443	-22%	-58%[1]

[1] 11-Year Change

Source: American Sports Data, Inc. -- SUPERSTUDY® of Sports Participation

Extreme vs. Traditional Sports

FREQUENT SPORTS PARTICIPANTS
AGES 6-24
(Thousands)

	6-11	12-17	18-24	25-34	35+	TOTAL
Team	6,500	9,805	3,874	2,607	3,680	26,466
Extreme	5,080	5,029	1,732	1,158	1,186	14,185
Outdoors	2,845	3,205	2,861	3,144	9,933	21,988
Fishing	2,360	1,976	1,944	2,462	6,305	15,047
Shooting	679	1,447	1,790	1,604	4,202	9,722
Racquet	508	1,170	851	517	2,306	5,406
Snow	767	1,064	655	570	1,337	4,393
Water	492	976	612	632	1,893	4,605

Source: American Sports Data, Inc. -- Sector Analysis Report

CHAPTER 23

THE STEREOTYPE OF "GENERATION Y"

"Generation Y" members, also known as "Millennials", "Generation Next", the "Echo Boom", or the "Digital Generation", were born (depending on the source) between 1977 - 1994, and are the latest issue of a genre that includes four other living cohorts: "Generation X" or "Baby Busters" (1965 - 1976); "Baby Boomers" (1946 - 1964); the "Silent Generation" (1933 - 1945); and the "World War II Generation", born before 1933.

Beyond the general contours of age, there is no precise (let alone empirically-derived) definition of these generational stereotypes; they are based on ascending proportions of fact, anecdote and fancy. While some of the defining behaviors (i.e. consumer purchases, health habits, suicide rates, etc.) are retrievable from the public record, the true essence of psychographic typologies -- personality, lifestyle, opinions, attitudes and social values -- remains largely undocumented, simply inferred by sociologists, trend-watchers, the media and other purveyors of popular culture. Generational typologies are merely demographics aspiring to psychographics.

No one can deny the existence of heavy metal, nose-rings, tattoos, and punk hairstyles; as a slice of Americana, Gen Y is real. But the vaunted typology -- itself fragmented into Goth, Skater, Surfer, Retro and other looks -- must share center stage with Hip

Hop, Preppy, Hipster and the dominant majority of more "conventional" youngsters.

A segmentation analysis performed by Teenage Research Unlimited, Inc. revealed that only 11% of the teen population occupies the "Edge" cluster -- a crude approximation of the Generation Y stereotype.

In many ways, "Generation Y" is a souped-up, improved version of "Generation X". Like its immediate predecessor, "Y" is laid-back, individualistic, resourceful, but also cynical; unlike "X", which was white/middle class/suburban, "Y" is socioeconomically, ethnically and sexually diverse. If sub-teens in the previous cohort were very advanced for their ages, Echo Boomers are dangerously precocious, an unsurprising characteristic of the most coddled and fawned-over children in history. Whereas "X"-ers were latchkey kids, "Y" returns from school to housekeepers; and if financial necessity forced many of the "Bust Generation" to live at home with parents, older Millennials are ensconced in their own apartments -- often subsidized by parents.

If "X" was contemptuous of authority, "Y" is downright inimical -- outrageously disrespectful to elders and constantly on the verge of a social coup d'état in which children will displace parents, teachers, employers and all other terrified dinosaurs of the old hierarchy. And while Millennials have mutilated the language even more horribly than did their Hippie ancestors -- they are the best-educated generation in American history.

The single greatest cultural achievement of "Generation Y" has been to expunge from our language the cherished pleasantry, "you're welcome" -- a time-honored utterance that once was the courteous, civilized response to "thank you". They have administered a multiple coup de grâce to propriety, civility and the mother tongue with a single linguistic bombshell: NO PROBLEM!!! And this verbal monstrosity (lexicographical masterpiece) is no longer a subtle defiance of politeness and conformity; it pervades every crack of the new lexicon, an all-purpose rejoinder to any statement imaginable!

Any member of the Silent Generation has borne witness to the parallel disintegration of authority, courtesy and the English language. Consider the evolution of a restaurant greeting, as an 18 year-old waitress seats a couple older than her grandparents:

- 1960: "Good Evening, Sir"
- 1975: "Hello, Folks"
- 1990: "Hi!"
- 1995: "H'ya guys doin'?"
- 2002: Her cell phone conversation interrupted, a distracted and annoyed waitress points to a table ten feet away and grunts the ultimate Millennial concession to politeness: "NO PROBLEM!!!"

While "Generation X" exhibited the highest rates of suicide, homicide, alcoholism, drug abuse, and pregnancy in teenage history, Millennials -- riding the coattails of a falling crime rate (easily the greatest unsolved mystery of the 20th century) -- have apparently reversed the trend. Quite inexplicably, this welcome reduction in teen misbehavior coexists with the Columbine stigma and a Millennial reputation for inwardly-focused aggression, substance abuse and generally antisocial behavior.

Not roundly criticized as slackers, "Y" kids are nonetheless characterized as apathetic, lazy and spoiled. But unlike "X" -- which was decidedly aimless, underemployed and pessimistic about its economic future -- "Generation Y" is pragmatic, worldly, materialistic, driven by technology and optimistic about its prospects. Indeed, if "X" was alienated and numbed, "Y" is very much alive, even passionate. There are signs of a paradoxical return to traditional values, most notably a renewed confidence in government leaders; and even more remarkably, a religious revival.

The technology-driven Millennial culture bears directly on its leisure preferences, especially participation in sports. "Boomers" were bred solely on network TV, while "Busters" added Cable, Atari and the PC to their repertoire. Millennials on the other hand, driven by email and the Internet, are able to detect emerging trends at virtually the speed of light -- a capability with enormous implications for the life cycles of fads and trends, both of which suffer serious time dilation. Brand loyalty and product preferences are also subject to change at hyperspeed -- a portent of even shorter product shelf-lives for sporting goods (especially footwear and apparel). The life spans of emerging sports are also potential casualties of time compression.

Torn jeans, inverted baseball caps, colored hair, nose rings, tattoos and stubble seem to proclaim an arrested state of emotional and intellectual development; but these are clever Millennial decoys -- symbols designed to conceal huge reserves of guile, determination, and a worldliness so keen as to cut to the very edge of paranoia.

The Stereotype of "Generation Y"

"Generation Y" has an inbred mistrust of major brands, resents obvious ad campaigns targeting their psychographic, and on the whole, poses a formidable challenge to all but the most astute teen marketers. Their razor-sharp defenses tolerate only the most subtle and "truthful" marketing messages; and these must be crafted by a copywriter who is indeed the supreme arbiter of "cool". But once the defenses of this super-savvy group are finally pierced -- as they have been by Tony Hawk, the 34 year-old cultural icon and one-man marketing phenomenon said to be the Michael Jordan of Skateboarding -- it can be a gigantic breach that invites the hordes of ESPN, Nickelodeon, The Simpsons, Interactive Video Games, films, CD's, books and a plethora of endorsements. It's only a matter of the right siege engine…and the degree to which Generation Y truly represents youth culture.

* * *

CHAPTER 24

THE GREAT OUTDOORS REVOLUTION: NEW LIFESTYLE OR STATE OF MIND?

FOR IMMEDIATE RELEASE   December 11, 2002

* * *

JEEPS, SAFARI VESTS, CAMOUFLAGE, HIKING BOOTS, AND CLIMBING WALLS DON'T ADD UP TO RUGGED OUTDOORS PARTICIPATION, STUDY FINDS

* * *

Camping and Hiking are flat, while only Artificial Wall Climbing and Kayaking Post Strong Recent Gains Amidst a Lackluster Outdoors Category

HARTSDALE, N.Y. -- It was hard-wired into our brains many thousands of years ago, and for millennia -- so long as the relatively few humans on the planet were one with nature -- it lay dormant and unnoticed. And it was only when they multiplied and became estranged from the environment that this instinct began to stir, finally taking root as the original conservationist ethic of the nineteenth century. The 1960's back-to-nature movement was the full flower of this longing, and a little later came the "green revolution". Today, our primal love of nature flourishes as a green blur of ecological awareness mixed with a growing appreciation of nature -- a blend symbolized by the insatiable demand for Outdoors fashion.

In the last few decades, consumer marketing has stalked this development, inventing and saturating us with "Rugged Chic" -- a staggering commercialization of the Outdoors theme that persuades beyond any doubt of an "Outdoors Revolution". But the so-called revolution is merely a state of mind, largely unrelated to rigorous participation in Outdoors activities. This conclusion was derived in part from the 15th annual SUPERSTUDY® of Sports Participation, conducted in January 2002 among 14,276 Americans nationwide, by American Sports Data, Inc. (ASD).

The proliferation of highly visible cultural symbols that have little to do with Rugged Outdoors participation -- Jeeps, Hummers, Parkas, Ski Jackets, Cargo Pants, Hiking Boots, Camouflage, Backpacks and Climbing Walls -- has elevated this fuzzy notion to dogma, almost above our ability to deny a Great Outdoors revival. On the other hand, abundant statistics document our passive bond with nature and the environment, but these only muddy the waters -- promoting the misconception that Americans are flocking to the outdoors.

While the number has declined from a decade earlier, in 1999, exactly one-half of all Americans (50%) considered themselves "environmentalists". According to the 2001 National Survey of Fishing, Hunting and Wildlife conducted by the U.S. Fish & Wildlife Service, in 2001 more than 66 million adults participated in feeding, observing and photographing wildlife -- up from 62.9 million in 1996. Since 1980, total recreational visits at national parks have increased by 27%... not a huge gain in view of population growth, but -- against the backdrop of declining overnight visits by Campers and Hikers -- suggestive of a healthy (if passive) interest in the Outdoors. A less salient (and perhaps less relevant) indicator of our growing Outdoors consciousness may be do-it-yourself home gardening among Americans -- which, according to the 2001 National Gardening Survey -- is at its highest level in five years.

But under higher magnification, the monolithic view breaks down -- revealing that over the past few years, the quintessential Outdoors activities of Hiking and Camping have either stagnated or declined. From 1998 - 2001, the number of Day Hikers in the U.S. dropped by 4% to 36.9 million, while Overnight Hiking/Backpacking fell from 6.8 million to 6.0 million participants, a drop of 12%.

During the same three-year period, Tent Camping -- the most popular Outdoors activity, grew by only 2%, to 43.5 million participants. The 19.1 million R.V. Campers projected in 2001 represent an increase of 5% over the 18.2 million measurement of 1998, but 16% below the 1987 estimate of 22.7 million. From 1980 - 2001, overnight R.V. Camping visits at national parks plunged from 4.4 million to 2.4 million. On the other hand, Tent Camping -- according to ASD survey research -- claims a 23% rise since 1987, but most of this growth can be attributed to population expansion. Over this 14-year period, <u>real</u> (per capita) gain for the activity would be about 7%. In 2001, overnight Tent Camping visits at national parks numbered only 3.3 million -- down from 3.9 million in 1980. During the same period, "Backcountry" overnight visits declined from 2.4 million to 2.0 million.

From 1990 - 2001, the number of "active" Outdoors enthusiasts (those who participated at least 15 days per year in at least one of the more rigorous activities -- excluding Camping) declined from 15.8 million to 15.3 million. Since 1998, the number of Mountain Bikers has plunged by 28% to 6.2 million, while the contingent of technical (rope and harness) Mountain/Rock Climbers has dropped 9% -- a statistically flat trend.

From 1998 - 2001, performance of the Outdoors sector is redeemed by strong gains in only two activities: Artificial Wall Climbing (+57%) and Kayaking (+35%).

Against the massive groundswell of public sentiment for environmental concerns, a growing affinity for nature, for wildlife and the Outdoors -- all of which are being fueled by the green revolution and authenticated by liberal consumer spending for Rugged outerwear, footwear and certain Camping products -- these lackluster Outdoors sports participation findings appear counterintuitive. But all too often, fashion trends and product sales have nothing to do with sports participation.

For example, by the late 1990's, after nearly two decades of the traditional "white shoe" look in athletic footwear, Americans were primed (if not desperate) for novelty. As a consequence, Hiking shoes, athletic leisure styles, sandals and brown casuals easily infiltrated the non-performance niche of athletic footwear, capturing the allegiance of bored consumers who had absolutely no intention of ever sweating in these new fashion offerings. As industry parlance studiously -- or innocently -- avoided the distinction between Hiking participation and Hiking shoe purchases, "Hiking" was soon decreed a trend.

In addition, record sales of backpacks had far more to do with schoolbooks and lunches than the Great Outdoors; and to a lesser extent, sleeping bags were purchased for sleepovers. But these artificial indicators of an Outdoors Revolution have been dwarfed by a colossal fashion statement provided by the Rugged Outdoor Apparel industry. While offering the same functionality that could have been satisfied by any number of mundane street styles -- heavy parkas, ski jackets, safari vests, cargo pants, farm overalls and camouflage transport the urban high-rise dweller to the tundra, jungle, desert, farm or any other natural habitat of his or her vicarious selection.

And in poetic affirmation of this ersatz Outdoors Revolution, Artificial Wall Climbing -- a decidedly indoor activity performed in climbing studios and upscale health clubs (where it is also mistaken for a fitness pursuit) -- has, as previously noted, registered a 57% participation gain from 1998 - 2001.

However, industry claims to record sales of high-performance products -- such as frigid-weather sleeping bags -- must be acknowledged; it is possible that a tiny, but flourishing "barkeater" segment of core Outdoors participants has simply gone undetected by the radar of large-scale population surveys. But even if this is true, survey research offers no comfort for those who cling to the myth of booming Outdoors participation trends.

The major disconnect between the new eco-consciousness and Outdoors participation is somewhat analogous to what has been observed of American attitudes toward physical fitness. Attitude and values change in the national psyche can be swift; but corresponding changes in behavior can be far less dramatic -- even glacial. ASD research has consistently shown that the vast majority of Americans (80%+) have already been persuaded of the virtues of physical fitness; yet only 20% are active fitness enthusiasts. Quite simply, our collective fitness behavior has kept pace with neither enlightened attitudes about the health benefits of fitness, nor symbolic identification with the fitness lifestyle. One is reminded of the decidedly overweight "Velour Runners" of the 1980's who donned elegant running suits with matching headbands, and expensive running shoes -- as they smoked incessantly on the sidelines of the New York City Marathon. Fitness folklore assures us that a good number of these emulators joined the growing army of fitness Walkers in the late 1980's; some later became joggers -- or in a few rare instances, marathoners.

The same dynamics and behavioral principles apply to

Outdoors sports/activities, where rigorous participation seems to lag a more generalized, but passive appreciation of nature and the environment. Following the well-established laws of human nature which urge us away from inconvenience, pain or discomfort (most notably the Pleasure Principle), the greatest numbers of people will opt for the paths of least resistance. Outdoors spectatorship (such as recreational visits to national/state parks) and light recreational involvement (bird-feeding, gardening, photography, walking) recruit the largest populations; less convenient forms of participation such as Camping attract smaller (but relatively large) followings, while the most rigorous pursuits (Hiking, Climbing) will claim the fewest devotees.

The Superstudy® of Sports Participation was conducted in January 2002 and based on a nationally representative sample of 14,276 people over the age of 6, who were among 25,000 respondents targeted in a sample drawn from the consumer mail panel of NFO Research, Inc. 103 sports and activities were measured along over 20 demographic, attitudinal and behavioral dimensions. Data were also collected on health club membership and other subjects pertinent to physical fitness. This annual tracking study has been conducted by ASD every year since 1987.

* * *

SELECTED OUTDOORS ACTIVITIES
Participated at least once
(000)
1998-2001

	1998	1999	2000	2001	3-Year Change 1998-2001
Artificial Wall Climbing	4,696	4,817	6,117	7,377	+57.1%
Kayaking	3,501	4,012	4,137	4,727	+35.0%
Trail Running	5,249	6,233	5,232	5,773	+10.0%
Camping (R.V.)	18,188	17,577	19,035	19,117	+ 5.1%*
Camping (Tent)	42,677	40,803	42,241	43,472	+ 1.9%*
Hiking (Day)	38,629	39,235	39,015	36,915	- 4.4%
Mountain/Rock Climbing	2,004	2,103	1,947	1,819	-9.2%*
Canoeing	13,615	12,785	13,134	12,044	-11.5%
Hiking (Overnight/Backpacking)	6,821	6,421	6,750	6,007	-11.9%
Rafting	5,570	5,000	4,941	4,580	-17.8%
Mountain Biking	8,611	7,849	7,854	6,189	-28.1%

* Statistically insignificant at 95% confidence level

SOURCE: AMERICAN SPORTS DATA, INC.

CHAPTER 25

SPORTS INJURIES: THE NEGLECTED STEPCHILD OF RESEARCH

MAGNITUDE OF SPORTS INJURIES IN THE UNITED STATES

Since 1987, American Sports Data, Inc. has been tracking sports and fitness participation in the U.S. In the year 2001, 50.6 million people over the age of 6 were frequent exercisers who participated in a single activity such as Running, Cycling or Treadmill exercise on at least 100 occasions. In addition, 39.9 million were frequent participants in a recreational sport such as Basketball, Tennis, Softball or Skateboarding, having participated at least 25 times, in most cases. Another 15.3 million were outdoors enthusiasts, engaging in an active outdoor pursuit such as Hiking, Mountain Biking, or Skiing, at least 15 times during the year. Many more Americans were less frequent players and participants; a clear majority of the population (68% or 170 million people) took part at least once in any of the sports/activities monitored by ASD.

A substantial number of these sports and exercise participants suffer injuries each year. Of the 35-40 million annual injury-related emergency room visits, approximately 10% are sports-induced -- an estimate confirmed in a pilot study of the present research which also indicated that less serious sports injuries (e.g. those not requiring ER treatment) -- were perhaps five times as numerous.

POTENTIAL GROWTH OF THE SPORTS INJURY POPULATION

Although no reliable tracking data can (as yet) affirm or deny this belief, sports injuries in the U.S. are becoming more and more prevalent -- across all age groups. While much has been written of late about a child obesity epidemic, the decline of Phys Ed in public schools, and the multitude of sedentary distractions that compete against the physical activity of children, there has also been a paradoxical increase in their sports injuries!

The contradiction however, is easily reconciled. First, while there has been a drop in traditional team sports participation among children, this fall-off has come from the less intense, unpressured, casual forms of pickup play -- which are in severe decline. By contrast, most organized team sports (except Baseball) have maintained participation levels, and a few, such as Soccer, Lacrosse and Fast-Pitch Softball -- may be flourishing. Unfortunately, the competitive culture of most <u>organized</u> youth sports is now so intense, it threatens not only the morale and character development of children, but their physical safety as well!

For reasons that may have something to do with the vicarious needs of parents, children are introduced to sports at unprecedented ages. Increasingly, children under the age of five are participating in Soccer, T-ball, Martial Arts and other sports -- practices that may also contribute to rising youth injury rates. A little later, the child may be forced to specialize; he or she may for example, be encouraged to play on three different Soccer teams, enduring three-hour practices, year-round. Naturally, this is a middle-class scenario; but sports and medical professionals sense that it is emblematic of the new super-competitive youth sports culture.

Sports Injuries: The Neglected Stepchild of Research

Youthful sports injuries are also being fueled by the increasingly popular non-traditional sector of Extreme Sports -- also dubbed "Millennial", "Alternative, or "Action Sports". An obvious argument is that extreme sports (Skateboarding, Snowboarding, Wakeboarding, Mountain Biking, etc.) are inherently risky and therefore conducive to rising injury rates; less obvious is the paradox that many children are driven by fanatical coaches and parents to the solitude and serenity of these more "dangerous" sports.

Baby Boomers (aged 35-54) continue to drive sports/exercise participation, and as a corollary, are generating higher rates of sports injury. According to the U.S. Consumer Products Safety Commission, sports-related ER injuries in this group increased by 33% from 1991 - 1998, but this rise -- according to CPSC -- paralleled increases in activity participation. Boomers are very important to the near-term future of sports medicine; many ushered in the original fitness movement and have made exercise a lifelong commitment. From 1987 - 2001, health club membership among people aged 35-54 increased by 135%; after stripping out the effect of population growth, the incidence of membership among this group could still claim a 60% rise.

The phenomenal growth of people over 55 in sports and fitness almost suggests an emerging branch of "geriatric sports medicine". From 1987 - 2001, health club membership of this cohort skyrocketed by 266%; and even after holding population growth constant, the increase was an astounding 219% -- clearly depicting a vast change in lifestyle and cultural values for older Americans. This trend is not limited to health clubs -- it extends to home/outdoors fitness, and also includes active recreational and outdoors sports. From 1990 - 1996, the CPSC recorded an increase of 54% in all sports injuries among people 65+ years of age; it also deduced from its data that sports and fitness participation is not limited to the youngest seniors. As the 65+ cohort ages, "they may remain active into their 70's, 80's and perhaps even 90's", a report states.

SPORTS INJURY EPIDEMIOLOGY:
A DEARTH OF NORMATIVE STATISTICS

Sports injury research is an intensely practical component of the sports participation knowledge base, and the mere existence of a sub-discipline called "sports injury epidemiology" (in this context, roughly the descriptive quantification of injuries deriving from sports participation) suggests a great abundance of vital data. But nothing could be further from reality: THERE HAS NEVER BEEN A MAJOR NATIONAL PUBLIC SURVEY OF SPORTS INJURIES IN THE U.S. -- at least not since the 1970's!

Given the considerable number and variety of groups that stand to benefit from such a research initiative, this is a curious state of affairs. Governing medical bodies, federal agencies, professional associations, educational institutions, municipalities and a host of other sports venues -- obvious beneficiaries of sports injury research -- should be natural evangelists for such an effort. Presumably, sporting goods manufacturers -- always fervent in the pursuit of safer products and protective equipment -- would also be eager consumers of such information; and not to mention the sports medical community, for which injury information is the very lifeblood. Then of course, there are a multitude of lower-profile users: federal agencies, safety groups, insurers, risk consultants, personal injury lawyers, etc. who are also natural beneficiaries. At the very least, we would expect that arbiters of sports medicine -- the de facto medical policemen who oversee research, publish journals, issue safety guidelines and other proclamations to the sports and fitness industries, might -- at some point or other -- have commissioned a national consumer study (counting all sports injuries, not just ER cases) on the very subject of their expertise. But not a single professional organization has made this effort!

CURRENT SOURCES OF SPORTS INJURY DATA

The general business of academe insures a continuous torrent of small-scale studies, dissertations and journal articles based on "local" data collection -- often single-sport inquiries involving small numbers of athletes on high-school or college teams. Perhaps an even greater volume of injury data is generated by the claims departments of insurance carriers; but this tonnage of proprietary data is highly confidential and highly focused -- compiled at the "micro" level on specific sports, situations, or recreational venues for the purpose of calculating product risk assessments, premiums, and many other actuarial functions.

At present, there are several large-scale injury surveillance systems, but not one provides a remotely accurate portrait of sports epidemiology in the U.S. Only one -- in the form of a public behavior study (but embedded as an afterthought in the National Health Interview Survey) -- is even capable of collecting nationwide "denominator" data. The ideal injury survey contains both "numerator" data (incidence of injuries) and "denominator" data (sports participation projections).

Other partial data sources are the following:
- NCAA Injury Surveillance System (ISS)
- Athletic Injury Monitoring System (AIMS)
- National Hospital Ambulatory Medical Care Survey (CDC)
- USCPSC -- National Electronic Injury Surveillance System (NEISS)

As the Holy Grail of sports injury data in the U.S., the latter study is invaluable; but it stands also as the national monument to a paucity of normative data on the subject. Based on a sample of roughly a hundred 24-hour emergency departments (in approximately 5,000 hospitals across the U.S.), the major limitation of this research is that by definition, it captures only relatively serious injuries...that is, only those requiring emergency room treatment. Preliminary data from the present study indicated that NEISS records only 15% - 20% of all U.S. sports injuries.

The second major flaw is that the CPSC estimates are based on injuries treated in hospital emergency rooms that patients say are <u>related</u> to products; it is therefore incorrect (according to a caveat in the report itself) to "say the injuries were caused by the product". In other words, the injury was not necessarily related to sports participation...as in the case of Dad tripping over a skateboard in the garage, or more disturbingly, a baseball bat used as an instrument of violence.

The weakest aspect of the CPSC study is its inability to render injury incidence or risk estimates, providing only what epidemiologists call the "numerator" -- e.g. the number of injuries. Since only a national survey of the U.S. population can furnish the total number of sports participants, (or derivative denominators), an emergency room study by definition precludes the necessary linkage between injuries, overall exposures, or more refined estimates of injury opportunity. Among its other shortcomings, NEISS has limited value for direct risk assessment; it cannot perform direct numerator/denominator calculations -- e.g. injuries per 100 sports participants, per 1,000 athlete exposures, etc.

POTENTIAL BENEFICIARIES OF INJURY RESEARCH

In principle, the loftiest purpose of injury research is to reduce the number and incidence of personal injuries that derive from sports participation; and since the 1970's, this has been achieved in certain sports by the introduction of rule changes, better protective equipment and safer products. As a boon to further progress, we must be able to gauge the overall magnitude and scope of the injury experience, and provide a descriptive analysis that can be used by epidemiologists, risk management consultants, academic researchers, product manufacturers, sports medical suppliers and all others who may strive toward the goals of injury treatment or prevention.

However difficult to imagine, sports injury research also has a potential commercial payoff: lower consumer prices of sporting goods and equipment. Aside from the alleviation of human suffering and obvious savings derived from unnecessary sports injury treatment, more accurate risk assessment for sporting good products and sports participation venues could result in lower liability insurance premiums for the insured -- a savings that presumably could be passed along to the end-users of sports products.

And this is not to mention the biggest potential bonanza: a safer image for sports, promoting increased participation.

Potential end-users of sports injury research include:
- Sporting Goods Product Manufacturers
- Insurance Carriers
- Protective Equipment Manufacturers
- Risk Management Consultants
- Sports Participation Venues
- Trial Lawyers
- Sports Spectatorship Facilities/Venues
- Sports Medicine Practitioners
- Sports Medical Equipment Supply Companies
- Sports Medicine Professional Associations

A COMPREHENSIVE STUDY OF SPORTS INJURIES IN THE U.S.

The present research is the first national "numerator/denominator" study since those conducted in the 1970's by Dr. Kenneth S. Clarke for the CPSC. The study is <u>unique</u> for three reasons:

1. It addresses the sports injury experience of <u>all people</u> over the age of six -- not just a sample of high school or college athletes, and is <u>projectable to the entire U.S. population</u>;

2. It addresses <u>all sports injuries</u> -- including less serious incidents and mishaps not requiring emergency treatment, left unrecorded by existing surveillance systems; and perhaps even more important, it monitors gradual/overuse injuries and conditions that are not sudden or traumatic, and therefore never treated in the ER -- but are often serious enough to require long-term therapy or even surgery.

3. It makes the direct connection between injury experience

and sports participation behavior -- i.e. the sample of injured athletes is drawn from the same sampling universe as sports participation behavior (<u>numerator and denominator derived from same sample</u>). The long-standing "apples and oranges" problem -- the inelegant, not to mention imprecise practice of divining injury rates by matching two completely different data sources -- is hereby eliminated.

As the definitive study of its kind in the U.S., the SUPERSTUDY® of Sports Participation has always offered a plethora of denominator data (measurements of 103 sports/activities and Health Club attendance) from its annual survey. In the January 2003 wave, a battery of Sports Injury items was added to the questionnaire:
- Sports Injury Experience
- Specific Type of Injury
- Sport/Activity
- Impact on Future Participation
- Circumstances of Injury
- Medical Treatment Received
- General Injury Type (Sudden/Gradual)

To enhance the analysis, injuries are classified according to degree of "severity":

LEVEL I
Injury did not interfere with subsequent participation.
LEVEL II
Injury prevented participation on at least one or more future occasions, but for less than a month.

Level III
>   Injury prevented participation for at least a month

Level IV
>   Injury prevented participation for at least a month <u>and</u> resulted in emergency room treatment, overnight hospital stay, surgery or ongoing physical therapy

Data will be presented both in aggregate form, i.e. <u>total</u> sports injuries and by individual sport/activity, including various (net) measurements. Analytical variables include demography, geography, injury severity, injury classification, (both general and specific), body area injured, medical treatment, participation consequences.

Sport-specific data are presented by number of participants, total athlete exposures, total number of injuries, incidence per 100 total participants, per 100 frequent participants, per 1,000 athlete exposures, by injury Level I, II, III or IV, major injury classification, medical treatment and impact on future participation.

* * *

CHAPTER 26

NEW NATIONAL STUDY IS FIRST SINCE 1970'S TO DOCUMENT FULL RANGE OF SPORTS INJURIES

FOR IMMEDIATE RELEASE   May 15, 2003

* * *

Sports Mishaps are Common -- But Less Than 1 in 5 Are Serious

* * *

Injury Rates for Most Extreme Sports and Exercise Activities are Relatively Low

* * *

Women Incur 40% of all Sports Injuries

HARTSDALE, N.Y. -- There may have been 20.3 million sports mishaps in the U.S. in 2002, but most were very minor: ankle twists, scrapes, bruises and jammed fingers accounted for a majority of these momentary setbacks. 11.2 million injuries (53%) were self-treated or remained untreated, while 6.1 million (30%) did not even hinder subsequent participation in the sport or activity. Only 3.4 million sports injuries were serious enough to require Emergency Room treatment. These were among the preliminary findings of a Comprehensive Study of Sports Injuries in the U.S., conducted by American Sports Data, Inc. (ASD) a Hartsdale, N.Y.-based firm specializing in sports and fitness research.

Because of their larger participant populations, Basketball, Running and Soccer yielded the highest number of injuries -- 2.8 million, 1.7 million and 1.6 million respectively. Not unexpectedly, Tackle Football had the highest injury rate in 2002 -- 18.8 per 100 players. "But on average, this means one injury every 5 player/years, and not necessarily a serious one at that," says ASD president Harvey Lauer. Ice Hockey, Boxing and Martial Arts have injury rates of 15.9%, 12.7% and 10.2% -- translating to just one injury every 6, 8 and 10 years, respectively. The annual rates of injury per 100 participants requiring ER treatment are lower: Football (6.1%); Hockey (6.6%); Boxing (11.5%); and Martial Arts (0.4%).

The most practical method of assessing risk potential in a sport is to measure the number of injuries per 1,000 athlete exposures -- i.e. the number of times a participant engages in the activity over the course of a year. Using this method, Boxing ranks first with 5.2 injuries per 1,000 exposures, followed by Tackle Football (3.8), Snowboarding (3.8), Ice Hockey (3.7), Alpine Skiing (3.0), Soccer (2.4), Softball (2.2) and Basketball (1.9).

With the exception of Snowboarding (which ranks third), none of the other so-called "Extreme" sports carries a particularly high risk of injury. Surfing is 10th in risk potential (1.8 injuries per 1,000 exposures); Mountain Biking 18th (1.2 per thousand); Skateboarding 22nd (0.8 per thousand); and BMX 24th, also with 0.8. In-Line Roller-Skating places 27th with only 0.4 injuries per 1,000 athlete exposures.

Sports Injuries in the U.S.

While membership in the "Extreme Sports" category implies a whiff of danger, only Paintball is handicapped by a huge injury taboo -- one that exists in the public mind, but not in the statistics. The industry has long maintained that the rare (but highly publicized) eye injury almost always occurs in an unsupervised, unprotected, often illegal setting; and that Paintball is a very safe activity -- a claim substantiated by the current research, as the sport reflected only 0.2 injuries per 1,000 exposures, the lowest injury rate of any Extreme Sport. Put another way, the average player will suffer a Paintball injury about once every 500 years.

40% of all sports injuries were incurred by women…an oblique and perhaps unwelcome confirmation of their near-parity with men in U.S. sports participation. And lest we chauvinistically presume that female injuries are somehow more benign, women also account for 37% of all ER sports injuries. In view of the strong female presence in Soccer, Volleyball and Cheerleading (all higher-risk activities) these findings are not surprising.

Children aged 6-17 represent only 19% of the 6+ population, but 38% of all sports injuries, and 46% of ER admissions. Boys in the 12-17 age group are the highest at-risk segment; with barely 5% of the population, they account for 17% of all sports injuries, and 23% of those requiring ER treatment.

The rate of injury for individual exercise activities appears extremely low. While Runners/Joggers racked up 1.7 million injuries in 2002, (a number surpassed only by Basketball), the incidence of Running injuries was relatively modest -- only 0.6 per 1,000 exposures, compared with 1.9 for Basketball and 3.8 for Snowboarding. Half of all running injuries (52%) were of the gradual/overuse variety -- not sudden/traumatic incidents.

Injuries resulting from equipment exercise were rare. Among those who trained with free weights or weight machines, 1.1 million were injured in 2002 -- an incidence of only 0.1 per 1,000 exposures. For Treadmill usage, the most popular form of cardio equipment exercise, the injury rate was also a microscopic 0.1 per 1,000 exposures. Even lower rates were found for Stationary Cycling and Stair-Climbing Machines.

A lower-than-expected injury rate appeared for Wrestling. With only 1.4 injuries per 1,000 athlete exposures, the sport placed 15th on this rigorous measure. Hunting registered only 0.8 per 1,000, for a ranking of 23rd. And in a not-too-surprising measurement, Softball was found to have a higher injury potential than Baseball -- 2.2 per 1,000 exposures versus 1.4 for Baseball. In Baseball, 63% of all injuries occurred in either the elbow (18%), shoulder (18%), knee (15%), or ankle (12%). For Softball, shoulder (17%), ankle (15%), knee (11%) and finger injuries (10%) accounted for 53% of the total. These data -- along with the specific injury descriptions reported by Baseball and Softball players -- strongly suggest that only a small percentage of all Baseball/Softball injuries are the result of a thrown or batted ball.

Sports Injuries in the U.S.

It has been widely assumed that for a variety of reasons, sports injury rates are skyrocketing; but overall trends in sports injuries are, according to Lauer, unknown. "For one thing, there hasn't been a dedicated national consumer survey done in nearly 30 years -- certainly not a 'numerator/denominator' study which addresses both injuries and sports participation in the same questionnaire," he said. By definition, the well-known emergency room study conducted by the Consumer Products Safety Commission documents only more serious sports injuries.

A Comprehensive Study of Sports Injuries in the U.S. is derived from the Superstudy® of Sports Participation, conducted in January 2003 and based on a nationally representative sample of 15,063 people over the age of 6 who were among 25,000 respondents targeted in a sample drawn from the consumer mail panel of NFO Research, Inc. 103 sports and activities were measured along over 20 demographic, attitudinal and behavioral dimensions. This annual tracking study has been conducted by ASD every year since 1987.

* * *

U.S. SPORTS INJURIES -- 2002
(TOP 25)

	TOTAL (000)	(%)	E.R. INJURIES (000)
TOTAL	20,145	100.0	3,358
Basketball	2,783	13.8	521
Running/Jogging	1,654	8.2	*
Soccer	1,634	8.1	259
Football (Tackle)	1,084	5.4	351
Softball	1,063	5.3	122
Strength Training	1,062	5.3	*
Volleyball	667	3.3	128
Football (Touch)	661	3.3	*
Martial Arts	610	3.0	*
Baseball	602	3.0	*
Fitness Walking	529	2.6	*
Bicycling (Recreational)	445	2.2	109
Tennis	415	2.1	*
Ice Hockey	415	2.1	171
Skateboarding	399	2.0	103
Walking (Recreational)	384	1.9	*
Cheerleading	323	1.6	*
Golf	291	1.4	*
Skiing (Downhill)	289	1.4	*
Aerobics (Net)	279	1.4	*
Horseback Riding	265	1.3	*
Roller Skating (In-Line)	252	1.3	105
Snowboarding	218	1.1	*
Hunting	207	1.0	103
Mountain Biking	201	1.0	*

* Less than 100,000

SOURCE: AMERICAN SPORTS DATA, INC.

CHAPTER 27

HUNTING, SHOOTING AND SOCIAL ANALYSIS

The refrain of social theorists has always been that the world is changing, and that the imprint of social change should be visible on all of life's major landscapes. If the observation post is high enough, the broad contours of social change are unmistakable: the world is becoming less formal, more casual, less authoritarian, but also less civil; at the same time, people are becoming kinder, gentler, and also smarter about their planet, their bodies, and their relationships with other living things.

If any of these lofty propositions are true, evidence of such truths should abound. We can test some of these hypotheses on various sports and fashion domains, beginning with the timely subjects of physical fitness, then proceeding to the most potent argument: hunting and shooting.

It is not an exaggeration to say that our national concern for health and fitness has reached epidemic proportions. The former proposition (that we are increasingly concerned about our bodies) is a good thing, and at first glance a resounding affirmation of social theory; the new fitness lifestyle seems to be a vote for humanistic evolution. But just as quickly, the idea of a fitness revolution is washed away by another highly-publicized megatrend -- the obesity epidemic.

We find a less ambiguous match between megatrends and sports in the fashion arena. Though they rarely witness perspiration, the ubiquity of warmup suits and athletic shoes are ringing testimonials to a less formal world -- but not necessarily to physical fitness. To complicate things just for an instant, formal dress-up is making a small comeback; but this minitrend poses no danger to the new casual milieu, and at least one aspect of our social theory appears vindicated.

Much less supportive of social theory is the near-lunatic behavior of a small percentage of parents and coaches at Little League, Hockey and Soccer games. This contradiction flies in the face of a kinder, gentler nation, leaving few traces of a more civil human condition.

Steroids use by celebrity athletes does not attest to a more enlightened world order; neither does the unrelated phenomenon of player/fan violence in professional Basketball. But these behaviors have nothing to do with sports participation, and derive from another megatrend: the massive collapse of authority and weakening of our social fabric.

By advancing female equality in sports participation, Title IX embraces the new humanism; but at the same time, opponents argue, the movement fosters intolerance and unfairness to male participants in certain secondary sports, (e.g. Wrestling and Gymnastics) who cry foul at the progress of Title IX toward the humanistic ideal of gender equity.

"Extreme Sports" such as Skateboarding, Snowboarding, Wakeboarding and BMX are solitary and decidedly antisocial; it can easily be argued that the major motivational ingredients of thrill, danger and the adrenaline rush are categorical advertisements for an angry, alienated youth culture which has no place in the new humanistic framework. But then, this youthful stereotype is not necessarily representative of the entire youth population.

So far, we have painted a blurred portrait of sports and social change; the relationship between sports participation and humanistic evolution has been less than unanimous.

What then of the Hunting and Shooting Sports? If ever there were a definitive microcosm of social change, we should find it here. In the capacity to enrage, enflame or simply stir the passions, no sports-related issue comes even close to the Shooting Sports drama -- in either magnitude or emotional volatility.

On issues of national importance, the collective impacts of all other sports issues and controversies can barely move the needle of public opinion -- much less influence a Presidential election. In 2000, Al Gore displayed too much fervor for Gun Control; in 2004, John Kerry -- until the last days of the campaign -- was too reticent in his affections for the Shooting Sports. Both were strategic blunders which may have altered the course of American history.

Shooting Sports in the U.S. are in severe decline. From 1987 - 2003, the number of Hunters plummeted from 25.2 million to 15.2 million -- a loss of 40%. Were it not for population growth, this fall would have been even more precipitous. Target

Shooting on the other hand has remained stable, edging up 4% during the same period. But if we consider the inexorable 1% annual growth of the U.S. population, this companion activity will also register a deficit, albeit one not so drastic (-11%). Civilian Handgun production and the issuance of Hunting licenses are by no means synonymous with trends in Hunting and Shooting; but neither do these "hard" statistics offer solace to the world of Shooting Sports.

In 2002, 14,996,406 Hunting licenses were sold in the 48 continental United States, down 10% from an aggregate 1975 tabulation of 16,597,807. The population-adjusted loss becomes (37%).

The trend in civilian firearms production between 1982 - 2001 is even less positive. Rifle and Shotgun manufacture in the U.S. have dropped by 21% and 23% respectively. Handgun production has suffered even more -- down 64% during the same period. On the other hand, some of these "losses" have been replaced by foreign imports, considerably improving the overall sales picture; but the net downtrend in both Hunting/Shooting sports participation is unmistakable. And contrary to Liberal nightmares, NRA membership -- though still a robust 3.4 million in 2003 -- had dwindled 20% from its peak of 4.3 million in 2000.

Armchair sociologists link the demise of Shooting Sports with the cascade of new social values spawned by the 1960's counterculture. But the problem is more complex, and like most social issues, defies quantification. Indeed, a wide array of forces -- most beyond its control -- militate against the industry. These include perceptions of rampant street crime and easy availability of weapons, a growing animal rights movement, highly-publicized school shootings, gun safety campaigns, a disappearing rural landscape, population trends, the cascade of kinder-gentler values and changing lifestyles, vanishing parental encouragement, competition from newer sports, and last but not least -- the seismic shift from outdoor to indoor recreation.

According to some observers, Hunting, Fishing, Trapping, Bullfighting, Boxing or any other activity with even the remote scent of a "blood sport" -- is swimming against the inexorable tide of humanistic evolution. The truly barbarous diversions of Cockfighting and Dogfighting have not yet followed into oblivion the ancient ritual of Bear-Baiting -- but they have been banished to arcane underground subcultures. In a far more humane context, the mainstream sport of Fishing -- with nearly 53 million participants -- is the top U.S. "blood sport", but it too has declined since 1987 (-9%). For a number of reasons, the "catch-and-release" method is gaining in popularity.

In addition, there are substantial legal, political and media assaults on the gun industry; but compared with the weight of public opinion and other societal trends, their collective injury is barely noticeable. Yet, the gun business survives; and if we believe more optimistic appraisals -- some Shooting Sports thrive! At a time when many trade shows are stagnating or withering, the premier industry trade event -- the S.H.O.T. show was the largest ever in 2004. Of course, the fortunes of a trade show can be unrelated to the vitality of its industry...

There remained in 2003, 28.5 million people over the age of 6 in the U.S. who participated at least once in any form of Hunting or Shooting with firearms -- a huge constituency, by any reckoning. ASD also finds that Hunting has a higher percentage of devotees than any other sport; in 2003, 32% of all Hunters claimed the activity as their "favorite".

The remarkable paradox of a thriving subculture "in decline" is best illustrated in a survey of 2,438 adult Americans conducted by ASD in July 2004. 82% agreed with the statement: "In general, I support the right of citizens to bear arms". This mandate is endorsed by a solid cross-section of the population, including 76% of all women, not to mention 68% of all Liberals, and -- somewhat astonishingly -- by 86% of Generation X. This lofty American value is far more than the quaint archaic bluster of an immature nation; it is embraced by 82% of all people holding Master's degrees, and is upheld across all economic strata and geographic regions. For most Americans, the "right to bear arms" is bedrock!

At the same time, Americans are intensely practical, recognizing that this monumental privilege is accompanied by an equally large responsibility. 9 out of 10 Americans (91%) agree that "people who buy guns should be required to report information about their backgrounds" -- an imperative that cuts across all demographic, economic and geographic lines. 88% of all Conservatives and 83% of all NRA members are in favor of background checks.

Interestingly, 13.8 million individuals were Handgun Target Shooters -- of which 8.9 million had no current interest in

Hunting, Shooting and Social Analysis

<u>Hunting participation</u>. It is conceivable -- though far from certain -- that this "secular" group of Handgun Users points to a new direction in the future of a declining Shooting Sports industry. Immune to the "blood sport" critique, these better-educated, upmarket individuals are motivated principally by Target Shooting and/or personal security concerns -- motives that cannot be assailed by humanists, animal rights activists or any other "ethical" objectors.

Which leads us to 9/11, and the generally accepted belief that the grotesquerie of that day spawned a profound global awareness of terrorism, and for indeterminate numbers during an indefinite period -- a frightful concern for personal safety and security. "Spikes" in retail gun sales and increased activity in background checks simmered in the aftermath of 9/11; but the terror was never absolutely linked to long-term public anxiety, the stockpiling of personal weapons, or to any other permanent aftermath.

A heightened concern for personal security could help shore up coffers in the coming years; but a more sporting and upbeat path to industry profitability may be Target Shooting. According to ASD, the vast majority of Americans (84%) regard Target Shooting as a "legitimate pastime, just like any other sport". This near-consensus spans the entire political spectrum: Liberals (81%), Moderates (87%), and Conservatives (83%).

With the abolition of Professional Boxing, the glacial footprint of humanistic evolution has been visible in Sweden since 1970. A similar prohibition has existed in China since 1949, but in both countries, the bans may soon be reversed -- major setbacks for evolution. In Portugal, the advent of the "bloodless" Bullfight is a step toward humanity, but one not sufficient to satisfy animal rights advocates.

In the U.S., the emerging sport of Paintball (a hybrid in which paint pellets are harmless substitutes for bullets) is one of the fastest-growing sports in the nation, advancing from 5.9 million players in 1998 to 9.8 million in 2003 -- a surge of 66%.

Sporting Clays -- or one of its descendants -- could be the ultimate Hunting/Shooting hybrid. With 3.9 million adherents in 2003, the sport has recorded a growth rate of 41% since 1998 -- the only Shooting Sport in positive territory, according to the ASD SUPERSTUDY®. This new blend, which allows mobile shooters to enjoy nature, and test their shotgun skills against a variety of simulated birds and animals (clay targets) hurled through the air or bounced across the ground, also enables participants to gratify their Hunting instincts -- without exposure to the ethical criticism or social stigmas arising from the wounding or killing of wildlife. The Shooting Sports may survive both its own extinction and the larger victory of humanistic evolution.

* * *

PART FOUR:
RESEARCH ISSUES

CHAPTER 28

ANALYSIS OF SPORTING GOODS MARKETS: THE PRIMACY OF SPORTS PARTICIPATION RESEARCH

Sports participation is generally the most powerful long-term predictor of market behavior in the sporting goods industry. In the short term, this postulate can be less reliable, and in some sectors, the connection between participation and product purchasing is at best, tenuous. There is a "hierarchy of correlation" between participation and purchases: in some instances, participation levels virtually <u>guarantee</u> higher product sales, while in others, absolutely no relationship exists between sport and product.

Axiomatic: Purchases for Participation

It is axiomatic -- but not certain -- that consumers participate in the activities for which they buy sporting goods and equipment. Snowboards are purchased for Snowboarding, Fishing Rods for Fishing, Baseball Bats for Baseball, and so on. For such activities -- after we smooth out the inconveniences of product durability, gratuitous fashion intervention, discretionary purchasing and the normal purchase cycle -- we should arrive, over a period of several years, at some confluence of participation levels and product purchases.

Some sports are more accommodating than others. Again, discounting inventory fluctuations, choked pipelines or other market vexations, we can expect -- even in the shorter term -- a fair congruence between Golf participation and Golf Ball sales, or between Paintball participation and paint sales.

Flies in the Ointment: Participation without Purchases

In many cases, people are not required to buy the instruments of sports participation; a good correlation between sports participation and market behavior can be spoiled by middlemen who pre-empt consumer purchases. Bowling Shoes, Skis and Paintball Markers are often rented; Treadmills, Weights and other exercise equipment may be used at Health Clubs, and Batting Helmets may be the property of teams, municipalities or school districts.

Axiomatic Reversal: Fashion Purchases without Participation

Fashion-driven athletic footwear and apparel markets are major exceptions to the sports participation/product purchase axiom. As ASD popularized 20 years ago, more than 80% of all "Running Shoes" are never sweated in, nor do millions of "Sweatpants" ever witness perspiration. Smaller exceptions to the rule are also found in the "Outdoors" market: most Backpacks are surely book bags, while many Sleeping Bags are merely purchased for "sleepovers".

In a different realm, a large percentage of firearms are destined neither for Hunting, nor even the Shooting Range…

The Raison-d'Être of Sports Participation Research

The general economy, industry conditions, product availability, fluctuations in discretionary income, and marketing campaigns all complicate the relationship between sports participation and purchase behavior. But at the end of the day (or at least at the end of several years) sports participation data generally correlate with longer-term market trends. Just as company "fundamentals" eventually decide market value at the micro-level, sports participation defines most sporting goods markets. In the final analysis, sports participation shapes the size, composition, and ultimately the product trend. Sports participation is in effect, the inexorable "gold standard" to which most markets eventually return.

The decline in Tennis participation since the early 1980's has closely mirrored shrinking levels of Racquet purchases, but a similar correlation between participation data and product purchases has not been found for Golf. According to ASD participation tracking research, even with the Tiger Woods-aided "blip" of 1997, Golf enjoyed only modest growth throughout the 1990's. However, these research findings were flatly contradicted by the mammoth gains of Golf product sales and industry stock prices during the same period.

Upon closer inspection, the phenomenal growth of certain Golf companies (most notably Callaway) was not attributable to any large expansion in the golfer population, but rather to the industry's genius for creating and successfully promoting newer and increasingly expensive products that elicited multiple "discretionary" purchases from an existing participant base. Exploiting the dream of every duffer to hit a Golf Ball farther and straighter, millions of Golfers who already had viable equipment were presented with a smorgasbord of space-age materials, vacuum cleaner-sized club heads, revolutionary new shallow-faced fairway woods and a host of other exotica they found irresistible. But toward the end of the decade, the over-priced, saturated Golf Club market experienced a screaming descent to reality -- one that should have been anticipated by the unremarkable growth of Golf participation.

Another example of sports participation research functioning as a "reality compass" was the sport of Fly-Fishing. From its inception in 1987 through 2001, ASD had consistently documented a shrinking Fly-Fishing population -- to the consternation and indignation of an industry convinced that their sport was enjoying remarkable growth. Industry opinion -- aided by the media, Hollywood, and the fervor of its participants -- had crystallized into an immutable "fact": that Fly-Fishing was one of the "fastest-growing" sports in the U.S.!

Unfortunately, precious little evidence (save the anecdotal) was ever produced in support of this thesis, and the competing view (based on participation research) was long unaccepted: that the population of Fly-Fishermen had been sinking, caught in the undertow of a general decline in overall Fishing participation. Depleted fish stocks, changing values, an evolving environmental consciousness, and competing leisure pursuits all militated against the growth of Fishing, which -- despite shrinking participation levels -- is still one of America's favorite pastimes.

In an entirely different arena, sports participation research was able to predict the demise of certain infomercial-driven Exercise Equipment -- years before a one-time darling of Wall Street was forced into bankruptcy. While the stock price of CML Group (parent of NordicTrack) soared, ASD research quietly revealed that Nordic Ski Machines were used predominantly in the home -- and not at Health Clubs. In the 1990's, this finding

The Primacy of Sport Participation

could have been corroborated by a visit to virtually any Health Club in the country. Many Clubs did not even have such a machine; and if one or two could be found, they invariably gathered dust on the Club floor -- a very clear signal that Nordic Ski Machines had failed the litmus test of Health Club acceptance. By contrast, Elliptical Motion Trainers, a rising star in the fitness firmament, register a much higher proportion of Health Club users -- a finding that validates the activity as an authentic trend. Unbeknownst to the investing public, the NordicTrack experience was confirming the old industry joke that "25% of all Home Exercise Equipment becomes a clothes horse within a month." Indeed, the skyrocketing sales of NordicTrack were ephemeral -- compliments of the once-omnipotent TV infomercial. Relevant point: this early-warning was sounded by a sports participation survey, and would not have been detected through standard product research.

On the positive side, for the past several years, ASD research has credited "senior" sports participation as a driving force in physical fitness and health club markets. This is not a forecast based on the well-known, burgeoning demographics promised by Census projections, but a proven historic sports participation trend. When combined with the explosive population projections for older demographics in the new Millennium, remarkably high fitness participation levels for people over 55 loom as the single most important finding ever produced by ASD -- an insight unattainable via any other form of sports research.

* * *

CHAPTER 29

INTERPRETING SPORTS PARTICIPATION RESEARCH

Sports participation statistics are of interest to a great number of individuals and organizations who regularly seek information on populations of sports participants: how many people play, how often, demographic profiles, geography, cross-participation, attitudes, motivations and other characteristics. These numbers -- both on individual participant sports or aggregate sector data -- find a wide variety of practical and theoretical applications: sporting goods market research, business plans, sports marketing surveys, health club research, exercise trend forecasting, public health assessments, sports injury epidemiology, tourism, advertising, and academic inquiries into the nature of cultural change are but a few examples.

Sports participation rates, physical fitness research and recreational trend data are found in daily newspapers, radio, TV, and now, on the most powerful information regenerator in history -- the Internet. Most often, the numbers are pursued and reported conscientiously -- with care and accuracy. Sometimes, the search and presentation is less fastidious; and on occasion, numbers are tweaked in support of a preconceived storyline. But very often, survey data are simply misunderstood or misinterpreted. There are five basic guidelines that govern sensible interpretation of survey research in the sports marketing context:

1. A Survey Is Not a Census

There are two ways of measuring sports participation behavior in the entire U.S. population: a complete census of all Americans, or a consumer survey which examines a representative sample of the population, and is able (with varying degrees of accuracy) to make reasonable estimates of its sports-related characteristics.

In an absolutely perfect world, the U.S. Department of Commerce would oblige ASD with a battery of sports participation questions added to the next Decennial Census. And if we accepted other Census imprecision, we might be able to state unequivocally for example, that there are exactly 34,857,014 Runners in the U.S., because we counted every single one.

But since a survey represents only a sample of a larger universe, it is subject to statistical uncertainty known as <u>sampling error</u>. This means that if 100 identical surveys (with the exact same format and questions) were conducted simultaneously throughout the U.S., the results of each would be somewhat different. But the differences would fall into a predictable range (larger sample sizes generally produce smaller differences) and we could talk about a "confidence level" associated with any or all of these surveys. Our limited resources allow only a survey in which one respondent in the sample represents 17,584 people on the ground, so we can offer only an estimate of 34,857,000 Runners that can vary by +/- 5.6% at the "95% confidence level." This means that if we've done everything else right (and leave aside other types of non-random survey bias), the odds are about 19-1 that there are somewhere between 32,905,000 and 36,809,000 Runners in the U.S.

2. To Be "Real," Year-to-Year Change Must Be Statistically Significant

If in 2003, two of only ten actual Americans interviewed across the country stated that they were Snowboarders, we could not -- with even a minute degree of confidence -- issue a news release declaring that 20% of the U.S. population participates in Snowboarding. If in the year 2004 (through a similarly futile exercise) we found that three of ten went Snowboarding, we could not proclaim that Snowboarding participation in the U.S. had jumped by 50% between 2003 - 2004.

Offending survey samples are not quite this insubstantial, but "trend" sightings in sports participation are often just as egregious. Companies and industry groups are eager to document "growth" in their sectors; the media are in perennial need of statistical validation for preordained news themes; and research providers, through a lack of rigor, patience (or even sophistication) seem to oblige with a remarkable aversion to significance testing.

Such abuses (often unwitting) are commonly illustrated in widely publicized surveys of 1,000 Americans, featuring the well-known, but often misleading +/-3% "margin of error". A survey of this magnitude may produce a grand total of 30-35 Snowboarders -- which may represent a "massive gain" of 50% over the prior year -- but which also happens to be statistically insignificant, and therefore only suggestive. While Snowboarding happens to be a "real" trend (with statistically significant change over time documented in larger surveys), growth in this activity cannot be proven here. In the same study, a 10% increase in a much larger activity such as Golf might be borderline at the 95% confidence level, not a "real" increase at all, and perhaps even the statistical equivalent of a 5% decline -- which might have been the result of an identical study conducted on the same day with a different sample.

For demographic sub-groups, the sample size requirements become even more demanding; we need larger samples to make reliable statements about "trends" for women in the 55+ age-group, or the Northeast, for example.

3. Different Methodologies Produce Widely Different Results

Even within the context of hardcopy mail panel research, tabulated results can differ tremendously between studies employing different methodologies.

1. Long questionnaires tend to produce respondent "fatigue" or "disinterest", while shorter questionnaires (particularly shorter sports/activities lists) produce higher sports participation projections.

2. Unduly long panel tenure can undermine respondent conscientiousness. Respondents who have been allowed to overstay their welcome on a consumer mail panel (when the panel has not been updated) generally exacerbate the "disinterest" factor, resulting in lower return rates, less fastidious questionnaire treatment and concomitantly, lower incidences of sport participation and purchases.

3. Low-cost omnibus questionnaires (where the head-of-household must collect data on all members of the household on a variety of subjects, always result in a smaller sports population. This unacceptable "economy" -- which allows

Interpreting Sports Participation Research

greater amounts of data to be collected at lower cost -- is the key difference between studies of American Sports Data, Inc. and the National Sporting Goods Association.

4. The presence or absence of a sport can make a great difference. My favorite example of amateurism: "Trail Running" was listed on a questionnaire measuring Outdoors participation, while regular "Running" was not. Purveyors of an egregiously inflated "Trail Running" projection had difficulty explaining it to the public. The subject is addressed at greater length elsewhere in this book.

4. All Sports Participants Are Not Equal

In 2001, according to ASD, there were 29.4 million people 6 years or older who played Golf at least once. This vast sport population forms a wide continuum of Golfers and so-called Golfers -- ranging from the reluctant duffer who played a single round on an obligatory business outing, to the retired zealot who lives in a Golf course condo, travels on Golf vacations, belongs to a private club and plays no fewer than 200 times a year. Yet both men enjoy equal status in the general participant population. Of our 29.4 million Golfers, 7.5 million (26%) played fewer than 4 times in the past year; 8.6 million played at least 25 times (an arbitrary definition of "frequent" golfer); and nearly 1.9 million (6%) spent over 100 days on the links.

Of 34.9 million "Runners," only 10.3 million logged in excess of 100 days during 2001, qualifying for the designation of "frequent" participant in this activity. 100 days of Running per year -- Herculean by Couch Potato standards -- is derided as minimalism by Serious Runners, who in addition to year-round training regimens of 30-50 miles per week, buy 4-5 pairs of running shoes per year, participate in road races/marathons, and subscribe to Running magazines. Whereas 6.4 million people ran on at least 150 occasions, (still not the province of elite athletes) the exclusive fraternity of "Serious Runners" numbers perhaps 2-3 million.

5. Analytically, Frequent Participants Are Surrogate Product Buyers

In general, roughly 20% of all participants in any sports or fitness activity constitute the core or "heavy users" of products and services. These dedicated amateur athletes are the backbone of the sporting goods industry -- representing a disproportionately high percentage of sales and repeat business. Very often, these "core participants" are market leaders and trendsetters emulated by the great mass of casual players. Analytically, <u>frequent sports enthusiasts are surrogate product buyers</u>. Using approximately the top quartile of participation frequency in each sport to define "core" participants, we usually find these groups to be excellent proxies for sporting goods customers -- both in demographic/psychographic profiles and absolute numbers.

For example, we can point to a rough equivalence between the 4.3 million frequent Soccer players (52+ days per year) and the combined memberships of USYSA, AYSO and SAY Soccer. A projection of 3.0 million frequent Baseball players (52+ days) dovetails neatly with an aggregate membership of 4 million in Little League, PONY, Babe Ruth and other major organizations. 3.5 million frequent Tennis players (25+ days) aligns with annual sales of roughly 4 million tennis racquets. Similarly, the estimate of 1.4 million frequent Skiers (15+ days) is consonant with the sale of a million pairs of skis; and in the same sphere,

Interpreting Sports Participation Research

1.2 million Snowboarders reflect the purchase of over a half million boards.

Marketers of athletic footwear, sporting goods, athletic apparel, and fitness products need to profile the sport's participants in order to understand the nuances of participation behavior. A knowledge of the <u>prime consumer</u> (Frequent Participant) is just as important as market share, price points, retail distribution and other sports marketing intelligence.

* * *

CHAPTER 30

SPORTS PARTICIPATION RESEARCH: NOT YET A SCIENCE

To paraphrase the famous comment on democracy, survey research is the very worst way to measure sports participation -- but it's the best one I've seen yet!

Sports Participation, when compared with the many bland topics of conventional marketing research (taste tests, shopping diaries, retail point-of-sale tabulations, etc.), is perceived as more interesting and entertaining to researchers and study populations alike; but while sports participation does have a certain appeal, its sexier subject matter confers no advantages on the research process. The rules and principles of sampling and question writing are governed by the same orthodoxies that rule more prosaic branches of research, and if pressed to name the first law of questionnaire design, ordinary researchers and sports researchers should both respond with the familiar imperative: "Ask people questions they can answer".

SPORTS PARTICIPATION -- THE METRIC OF CHOICE

Dollar sales volume -- as in a $61 billion soft drink market, $183 billion prescription drug sector or $8.6 billion cell phone market -- is a popular way of depicting the magnitude of a product. In some categories, markets are more vividly portrayed by participation behavior. 85 million gardening households, 159,000 professional photographers, 32 million crossword puzzle aficionados or 50 million frequent fitness participants are handy statistics -- for some purposes, more valuable than fragmented, indecipherable purchase data which lack context. When products are consumed on a frequent basis, or by nearly everyone, it often makes sense to think about the size of a market or industry volumetrically -- by product units rather than people. Hence, annual U.S. consumption of 1.5 billion gallons of orange juice is arguably more utilitarian than say, a near-unanimity of 250 million orange juice drinkers.

In the sporting goods industry, markets are usually described in terms of participation behavior. While the number of Baseball bats, gloves, and helmets are indispensable statistics, one hears more often about the population of 11 million Baseball <u>players</u> -- not about the equally important measurement of product purchases. On the other hand, the U.S. athletic shoe market is not readily captured by sports participants, because they represent only a minority of buyers; as I popularized twenty years ago, 80% of all athletic/sports shoes are never sweated in. But this is another matter.

In sports participation, the convention is to describe a population in terms of 12 million Beach Volleyball players, not as a volumetric behavioral estimate of what might be called "tonnage" -- e.g. 271 million aggregate national participation days or Volleyball experiences per year. Tonnage is often a more precise measure of sports participation, but too awkward for practical usage. Marketing professionals have difficulty operationalizing "2.6 billion aggregate Running days in 2002"; cognitively, 36 million Runners is a far more riveting and actionable metric, translating easily into demographics, products and markets.

Sports Participation Research: Not Yet a Science

WHO IS A "PLAYER"?

To discover the approximate number of Baseball players, Gymnasts or Stationary Cyclists in the U.S., we need to define "player" or participant; we then conduct a survey of the entire population. It is not sufficient to ask whether or not respondents "play Baseball", regard themselves as "Billiards players", or claim to be "Surfers"; at best, subjective self-descriptions are loose and imprecise. A second convention is to define a sport/activity participant (e.g. Treadmill user, Yoga practitioner or Lacrosse player, etc.) as someone who participated in the activity <u>at least once in the last 12 months</u>. Aside from the relative handful of respondents who may have participated in a sport only once or twice about a year ago, this question is neither daunting nor freighted with ambiguity. If all else goes well, such straightforward queries (requiring even 12-month recall) produce viable measurements of sports populations. Most of us know if we Bowled at least once in the past year, or did <u>not</u>; if we Ran at least once, or did <u>not</u>, etc.

THE "TELESCOPING" PROBLEM

Still, minor distortions are inescapable, even for simple measurements of sports participation. A small number of respondents succumb to "telescoping" -- incorrectly recalling for example, that a single, isolated Bowling night 15 months ago happened within the "last 12 months". Or perhaps the person does remember the exact date of the "non-qualifying" Bowling experience... but that it occurred outside the 12-month time-frame is utterly beside the point; <u>he or she simply wants credit for it</u>!

<u>Occasional</u> sports participants are more susceptible to telescoping, and therefore are more likely to artificially inflate the measurement of sports populations. Sports that are played or participated in less often (e.g. Skiing, Scuba Diving, etc.) are at *higher risk* for this type of distortion than say, Running or Walking -- sports/activities that are indulged in more frequently. This is because occasional or infrequent participants -- the "at-risk" groups -- constitute a larger proportion of "smaller" sports, and a smaller percentage of "larger" sport populations.

In 2002 for example, a majority of the 3.3 million projected Scuba Divers engaged in that activity fewer than four times, suggesting a high potential for inflated measurement -- *if* the dates of some occasional experiences (which occurred more than a year ago) are incorrectly reported. While rare events are more salient and easier to date -- especially when they happen on a winter vacation, or during some other particularly memorable time -- there is little doubt that certain of these distinctive experiences are deliberately misplaced in time (included in the 12-month recall period).

From this point of view, telescoping is less vexing in higher-frequency sports and activities. Only 5% of our 35.9 million Runners participated fewer than four times; 63% ran more than 25 times. It would seem therefore, that whether or not one has run "at least once" in the last year is a less challenging cognitive task -- and also one that invites less dissembling. Most alleged "Runners" are truly Runners.

Sports Participation Research: Not Yet a Science

Memorable sports participation <u>events</u> may be even more susceptible to the telescoping of time -- even though the amateur athlete can accurately date such occasions. Very often, a marathon run 18 months ago will, in the mind of the respondent, have occurred within "the last 12 months". This is not memory distortion at a preconscious level, but far more often, a simple conscious desire to receive credit for a prodigious athletic feat...and precisely when it happened is totally irrelevant! Once again truth becomes a casualty, and unsuspecting consumer researchers who measure "marathons" or "triathlons" will be astonished at inexplicably large numbers...

ANTIDOTES TO TELESCOPING: SPURIOUS OR UNAVAILABLE

Critics of sports participation research point to the difficulty, if not futility of 12-month recall; is it not absurd to think that a person might accurately recall the number of times he or she has Skied, Golfed, or visited a Health Club in the last 12 months? A solution they argue, is a three-part question: number of days per week; number of weeks per month; number of months per year. Here, computerized multiplication improves on the respondent's hasty calculations and scribbled margin notes, ostensibly providing a more "accurate" estimate. But in the end, this "refinement" confers no material advantage: the result will be an inflated number -- similar to the respondent's answer to a single open-ended question about the "last 12 months".

In a noble but misguided effort to side-step long recall periods, undergraduates in sports management courses (and all too many professional researchers) innocently ask: "how many times <u>per week</u> do you participate in".....This approach discounts seasonal, sporadic, or occasional participation, and assumes the respondent is a 52-week year-round participant who faithfully adheres to a weekly regimen. Needless to add, such data are worthless.

On occasion, when abundant resources have permitted more frequent surveys and compacted research periods (e.g. monthly, weekly or even daily surveys) members of the general research community innocently believed they had finally outwitted 12-month recall. By simply adding the daily, weekly or monthly results of these more frequent surveys with shorter recall periods, they have blissfully -- and quite naively -- "discovered" the Holy Grail of accurate, annual sports participation projections.

This is a staggering failure of logic. We cannot merely sum 12 individual months, 52 individual weeks, or 365 individual days of independently surveyed sports participation and arrive at an annual grand total; any such aggregation will <u>always exceed</u> the true number. Twelve monthly surveys of Basketball players cannot be added for an estimate of how many people played the sport in the past 12 months -- without double-counting! The simplest illustration: If there were two days in a year and three people in the U.S. (one of whom had biked on both days, another on one day, and the third not at all), there would obviously be <u>two</u> cyclists in this miniature nation -- a result obtainable <u>only</u> through an <u>annual</u> survey asking about <u>any</u> cycling activity throughout the <u>entire</u> (two-day) year. A survey conducted for Day 1 (showing <u>two</u> cyclists) added to an independent survey of Day 2 (showing <u>one</u> cyclist) will fallaciously yield three cyclists -- not the *true* "population" of <u>two</u> cyclists.

Sports Participation Research: Not Yet a Science

	Day 1	Day 2	Days	Cyclists
Person A	√	√	2	1
Person B	√	0	1	1
Person C	0	0	0	0
	2 +	1 =	3	2

It would be permissible to add <u>volumes</u> of products -- such as the total pairs of athletic shoes purchased or total gallons of orange juice consumed. <u>But we cannot add periodic shoe buyers, orange juice drinkers, or Runners to arrive at annual totals</u>.

FREQUENCY OF PARTICIPATION -- OVERSTATED, BUT USABLE

Telescoping, to varying degrees, will result in the artificial elevation of <u>sports populations</u> -- how many people <u>participate</u> in a sport; but for the bigger sports, these overstatements are not significant. Far more serious exaggerations occur in self-reports of <u>participation frequency</u> -- how *often* people play or engage in a sport/activity, usually in *days (times) per year*. Memory is quite fallible, and in most behavioral measurements -- certainly in the case of sports participation -- humans tend to err on the high side. Unless we have the luxury of a daily consumer diary, the recall problem -- be it innocent memory distortion or deliberate dissimulation -- cannot be avoided.

Respondents are quite consistent in <u>overestimates</u> of total sports participation days, which are usually much higher than "objectively" derived measures from lift-ticket sales at Ski resorts, card-swipes at Health Clubs, or register receipts of daily fees at public Golf courses. On the other hand, these more "objective" nose counts -- for a multitude of reasons -- are never useful in projecting the size of a sports population. For example, the entire universe of Ski areas might not be captured (or known); informal, off-site participation (e.g. in Paintball, Ice-Skating, Snowboarding, etc.) may be huge; gratis, non-paying seniors may go uncounted; Bowlers may own, not rent shoes; people may hunt or fish without licenses, etc. Virtually any market or product-based data compilation will fall short of the Divine Truth.

In 2004, the crude and inexact method of consumer recall is the only practical methodology with which to gauge aggregate sports participation behavior on a national scale. Bloated results cannot be adjudicated by weighting procedures, and the only form of damage control is an awareness that "average number of participation days" (not total number of participants) are likely overstated 20% - 50%, across-the-board, regardless of research method. In very long self-administered surveys -- where, for a very different reason, the total numbers of participants are underestimated -- there may be a serendipitous cancellation effect, accidentally producing a more "accurate" projection of sports participation.

For aggregate sports participation (persons multiplied by number of days), the Golden Mean lies somewhere between the extremes of survey research and various forms of industry or product-based reckoning.

THE EFFECT OF TELESCOPING: A UNIQUE QUANTIFICATION

The National Human Activity Pattern Survey (NHAPS), conducted by the Survey Research Center at the University of

Sports Participation Research: Not Yet a Science

Maryland from October 1992 - September 1994, provides a rare opportunity to gauge the extent of telescoping. NHAPS interviewed 7,515 adults on a daily basis, employing a 24-hour recall methodology. Respondents were asked to enumerate each and every activity (e.g. sleeping, eating, driving, exercise, etc.) performed on the previous day. The research objective was to quantify total energy expenditure by Americans, with activity categories taken from a "Compendium of Physical Activities", developed at the University of Minnesota. The data were then assiduously coded and converted into aggregate units of energy. This landmark research has not been replicated, but its 24-hour recall methodology remains a unique standard for assessing the effects of telescoping in sports participation research.

Unfortunately, the NHAPS study delineated only a handful of specific sports/activities, such as Basketball, Bowling, Tennis, etc. The vast majority of sports and activities were lost to either compound measurements (e.g. Fishing/Hunting), or miscellaneous aggregate categories, such as "Other heavy sports/exercise". In the end, only 5 meaningful comparisons could be made with ASD participation data from approximately the same period.

If we accept NHAPS as the gold standard, redemption for 12-month recall is at hand only for Golf. Over a two-year period, 63 of the 7,515 adult respondents reported playing Golf on the previous day. This microscopic daily average Golf participation (.0084), when multiplied by the 1993 U.S. adult population of 185.4 million, yields an <u>average</u> of 1,557,360 Golfers playing on any single day. This figure, multiplied by 365 days per year, results in an aggregate 568,305,000 total player/days, the only comfort for an independent 12-month recall comparison -- approximating 582,806,000 aggregate Golf days projected by ASD for 1993. This unusual and inexplicably accurate Golf recall has been noticed elsewhere, and the only plausible explanation is tongue-and-cheek: Golfers are more likely than any other sports participants to repress painful memories -- thereby reporting fewer outings, and as a corollary, attenuating the telescoping problem!

The five available comparisons between ASD and NHAPS data were the following:

AGGREGATE ADULT PARTICIPATION DAYS (1993)

	ASD (12-month recall)	NHAPS (24-hour recall)	Telescoping Effect
Golf	582,806,000	568,305,000	+ 3%
Tennis	282,582,000	209,780,100	+35%
Bowling	507,656,000	297,752,400	+70%
Soccer	145,389,000	108,273,600	+34%
Basketball	633,120,000	331,587,900	+91%

RESPONDENT RECOGNITION: THE NEED TO BE "INCLUDED"

It is axiomatic that people want to be recognized for athletic achievements. This is true not only for high-school swim records, college football rosters, or later-in-life 5K race times, but for mundane sports/fitness participation of no particular moment, except to the respondent who, quite understandably, is determined to inscribe these personal achievements in the annals of sports research. In a survey of Outdoors sports participation, a well-known research firm momentarily rocked the sporting goods industry with a "discovery" of over 50 million "Trail Runners"! This absurdity was the result of a fatal omission: along with the standard list of Outdoors sports and activities such as Hiking, Camping and Canoeing, the hapless questionnaire writer dutifully included "Trail Running" -- but not "Running"! Ninety percent of the resultant "Trail Runners" were mere frustrated Road Runners who simply needed recognition for participation, choosing to sublimate pent up mental energy through the only available outlet in the survey instrument -- Trail Running. By contrast, American Sports Data, Inc. projected a far more reasonable number (only 5.6 million Trail Runners for 2002), and of course, many, many, more Road Runners.

MAN-MADE OBSTACLES: LONG QUESTION BATTERIES
Were there really 55 million Bowlers in 2003, as proclaimed by American Sports Data, Inc.? The answer -- quite apart from the universal issue of random but predictable fluctuations due to sample size -- is that consumer mail panel research (like quantum physics, which tolerates the ambiguity of an electron -- or anything else -- in two places at the same time) allows both more and less than 55 million Bowlers.

Due to simple respondent fatigue, or more dangerously, waning interest in panel membership, long lists of sports/activities ensure lower response rates -- more so for sports appearing at the ends of long batteries. Even if we reverse the order of presentation for half the sample, the problem is attenuated, but not solved completely; any self-administered questionnaire battery in excess of 25-30 line items will understate whatever is being measured. But there is a counterweight -- the telescoping effect will artificially <u>add</u> sports participants, restoring some of the deficit.

On the other hand, statistics derived from single questions are somewhat more immune to respondent fatigue or disinterest. For example, the ASD projection of Health Club membership (based on a single stand-alone question), aligns closely with other (triangulated) approaches; and this confluence of independent findings provides much comfort. Shorter batteries (or individual questions) generally produce higher sports participation estimates.

THE MOST TREACHEROUS PITFALL: BORED, DISINTERESTED PANELISTS

This problem is endemic only to consumer mail panel methodology, and is treated at length elsewhere. As we know, nothing is free, and the tremendous cost savings of consumer mail panel research (elimination of the interviewer) exacts a huge tradeoff: unreliable response patterns from panel members who have outlived their usefulness.

Known in the trade as "Eager Beavers", newly minted panelists faithfully execute their duties with care and precision, generally producing higher rates of sports participation (or any other behavior) than longer-tenured respondents. Fresh recruits tend to be diligent and conscientious in filling out questionnaires; but whether or not Eager Beavers reflect the ultimate "true" reality may never be known. It is conceivable that these bright-eyed novices actually over-report sports participation behavior.

Indeed, recently recruited panel members -- according to experimental research conducted by ASD in 1997 -- reflected sports participation rates 22% higher than those of more seasoned panelists. Even less comforting was the perfect negative correlation between tenure and incidence of sports participation: with each successive year of panel membership, respondents became less attentive and fastidious to questionnaire completion -- a trend paralleled by eroding sports participation rates, known as the "Lazy Dog" effect. Age contributes somewhat to the variance.

Panel Tenure		Sports Participation Rate
<1 year	=	100% -- Benchmark
1-2 years	=	91%
2-3 years	=	88%
3+ years	=	82%

Great care must be taken to ensure that each year, the final sample contains roughly similar proportions of panel members in various stages of the membership cycle. This can be accomplished via sample weighting, where panel membership tenure is treated as an additional variable in the sample balancing program.

The failure to account for changing tenure composition in consumer mail panels can be fatal -- producing unaccountable fluctuations in year-to-year tracking results.

RESPONDENT COOPERATION:
SMARTER QUESTIONS, BETTER ANSWERS

A recent government-sponsored study offered the "illumination" that 82% of Americans aged 16+ (175 million people) "walked" at least once in the past year! This profoundly useless statistic is undoubtedly correct, but has approximately the same zero value as a national estimate of "exercisers" or the number of people "active in sports and recreation".

When questionnaires clearly define a sport or activity, people reward such detailed painstaking nomenclature with more relevant, actionable results. For example, a three-pronged measurement of Court, Grass and Beach Volleyball is far more sensible than a one-dimensional estimate of Volleyball. Over the years, the American Sports Data, Inc. SUPERSTUDY® of Sports Participation has made similar refinements to the line-item definitions of Tackle Football, Wrestling, Mountain Climbing, Bicycling, Swimming and many others. An original measurement of "Football" may have yielded 21 million players, and then, cinched by a more rigorous definition of "Tackle Football", narrowed to 10 million. With the ultimate refinement of "protective equipment", the number was halved to a more realistic estimate of only 5 million.

RESPONSE DISTORTION: A BRIEF SUMMARY

The telescoping of time is usually a form of preconscious memory distortion. Sometimes it is deliberate and conscious; people simply *want credit for activity performed more than a year ago* -- or in rare cases, for activities never performed at all. Another type of response distortion is driven by simple ego-need: the tendency to present ourselves in the most flattering light and to inflate our achievements…in this case *to exaggerate the number of participation days* we report. People also need to *feel "included"* in a survey -- especially when one of their sports is missing from the questionnaire. On occasion, they may actually <u>forget</u> some instances of participation, but this is rare. More commonly, research subjects, especially in mail surveys, may -- for reasons unrelated to memory capacity but very much associated with lackadaisical attitudes toward the interview or a widening alienation from panel membership -- simply fail to report participation in various sports and activities.

BOTTOM LINE: WHAT CAN WE TAKE TO THE BANK?

Without the cooperation of the Census Bureau, the divination of sports participation (or any national statistic) becomes exceedingly difficult, because research -- subject not only to the vagaries of random sampling error -- must negotiate other minefields. In general, five problems afflict sports participation research:

- Panel Tenure (Understates Sports Participation)
- Questionnaire Length (Understates Sports Participation)
- Telescoping (Overstates Sports Participation)
- Forgetting (Understates Sports Participation) -- Rare
- Poorly Defined Sports Categories (Various Impacts)

Burnt-out panel members will artificially depress sports participation projections, as will unduly long question batteries. Telescoping has the opposite effect, but it almost certainly does not entirely compensate for losses exacted by bored respondents or oppressive questionnaires. An educated guess is that with proper weighting procedures and reasonable questionnaire length, the results of a mail panel study will not differ greatly from similar surveys conducted with other methodologies.

We will never know the precise count of Wakeboarders or Pilates practitioners, but basically sound (if crude) methodologies are able to capture the general magnitude of a sport population. More important, consistent year-to-year methodologies can provide very accurate trending.

Due to other sources of measurement error, we know that even a Census count of Skateboarders or Mountain Bikers could not be engraved in stone. But through a "triangulation" of measurements from various other consumer surveys, magazine readership, industry product market estimates, obligatory governmental tabulations and other external sources, we know that survey research can produce national projections of <u>high face validity</u>.

The case for confirmation is strong. The 2002 ASD projection of 51.4 million Fishermen exceeds, but is perfectly consonant with the roughly 28 million Fishing licenses sold each year in the U.S. With the application of a little "Kentucky Windage" the estimate of 36 million Health Club members across the U.S. (18 million of whom are "Commercial" Health Club members) is gratifyingly close to a nationwide Yellow Pages compilation by InfoUSA. For over 15 years, ASD Health Club membership trends derived from consumer research has accurately tracked "known" Health Club expansion (supply quickly catches up with demand), as gauged by this independent service. The ASD finding of 4.1 million frequent Soccer players is an excellent proxy for the combined memberships of USYSA, AYSO and SAY Soccer. About 15 million Hunting licenses are issued each year by the 50 states…a number which dovetails neatly with 16 million Hunters projected by ASD (licenses are more obligatory in

Hunting than Fishing). In addition, for Outdoors sports participation, the periodic U.S. Fish and Wildlife survey produces results very similar to those provided by ASD. To the best of our determination, the Tennis industry sells roughly four million tennis racquets every year -- a not unreasonable contrast with the ASD estimate of 4.0 million <u>frequent</u> Tennis players in 2002.

THE IMPERFECT SCIENCE: SOLUTIONS FROM A PERFECT FUTURE

By the year 2050, technological progress will have taken us far beyond our quaint reliance on fallible human memory and perception. Unobtrusive monitoring devices -- gleaning data from bodily implants, or perhaps even less obtrusive retinal scanning devices -- will free respondents from the primitive need to remember "how many days per year"...Investigators of sports participation behavior will avoid the minefield of consumer research altogether, because hard physiological data will have finally trumped soft social science.

* * *

CHAPTER 31

POINT-OF-SALE (POS) RESEARCH IN THE SPORTING GOODS INDUSTRY

In theory, point-of-sale (POS) research is a superior source of marketing information that offers a high degree of accuracy for whatever product data are captured. The process begins at the retail counter, where impersonal barcode scanning circumvents the weaknesses of consumer research.

POS research is not error-free, but barcode scanning does ensure fairly precise reporting and tabulation of category, price, retail distribution channel, brand, model, size and other encoded product information. Totally objective computerization avoids the frailties of human reporting, exempting POS research from criticisms leveled against methodologies based on the respondent's memory of a purchase experience. Consumer research surveys can be invaluable, but memory-based reporting (even a daily diary) is subject to various forms of conscious and unconscious distortion: forgetting, "telescoping", boredom, fatigue, disinterest, carelessness, or simply the need to be "included" in a survey.

On the other hand, while POS research generally claims high-grade accuracy, such studies (with rare, futuristic exceptions) don't tell us anything about the buyer at the cash register. Consumer surveys by contrast, can provide an endless array of demographics, psychographics, product usage, sports participation, attitudes, health habits and other consumer behavior -- in addition to the core marketing elements of category, price, channel and brand. If done properly, a consumer survey is also projectable to the entire market or population; as a practical matter, the POS study is not.

But the really prohibitive problem with most POS studies is that they <u>do not generally represent all retail distribution channels</u>, and even more seriously -- due to a lack of respondent cooperation -- <u>cannot even adequately sample part of a given distribution channel</u>.

A well-known industry study exemplifies both deficiencies. Its data collection points (retail stores) include Kmart but not Wal-Mart; JC Penney but not Sears; Footaction but not Foot Locker, etc. Even worse, the paucity of Specialty retailers is a gigantic black hole: Exercise Equipment, Golf Pros, Bicycle Stores, Gun Dealers and Ski Shops -- among other specialty outlets -- are poorly (if at all) represented. <u>In such a study, the greater the importance of the specialty retailer, the greater the distortion of brand share and all other reported data</u>. Conversely, industries with a heavy reliance on mass merchants and discount stores (athletic footwear and camping, for example) may find a vaguely realistic portrait of the marketplace. But in Golf, a category heavily vested in Specialty channels, Callaway -- the undisputed market leader -- is inexplicably absent from the top brand rankings.

In addition, only a small fraction of all Sporting Goods categories are addressed, and among those measured, product breakdowns are vague or insufficient.

Point-of-Sale Research

Some years ago, a POS study of Specialty Retailers in Sporting Goods had the opposite problem: it emphasized smaller retailers at the expense of large chains, and was further handicapped by a geographically skewed distribution of stores dominated by the northeast.

Yet for all these deficiencies (and laying no claim to a sample weighting scheme!), POS studies purport to measure "brand share", "total size of market" and "top sellers". In reality, actual market volume may be several times that depicted for most categories, while no single market is <u>accurately</u> portrayed.

To make matters worse, unmodulated year-to-year "comparative" data are typically shown without any adjustment for new stores added in the current period. Naturally, a fair contrast with the prior year must show "same store" comparisons -- but methodological propriety is rarely a concern of the POS research entrepreneur.

On the positive side, any designer of syndicated research appreciates the brute labor and painstaking effort demanded by such a gargantuan project...and can only applaud the effort. But at present, POS research is based on a large, amorphous chunk of the market -- an undefined fragment of the retail universe. Tabulations of a partial, indescribable, constantly changing sample will be misleading -- especially when misinterpreted as representing the <u>entire</u> sporting goods market, or even an individual category. A POS study can never divine the true market share of Reebok, the number of Mountain Bikes sold through discounters or how many dozen Golf Balls were purchased at Pro

Shops -- much less across the entire U.S.

The results of a POS study (in theory) can be legitimately presented in one of two ways -- but neither one is feasible. The first remedy is to vastly increase the scope of research coverage by enlisting near-perfect retailer cooperation in all product categories. The second is to somehow weight the raw data, projecting it to a known retail universe. Unfortunately, the complexities and uncertainties of the latter option are incredibly daunting, if not insurmountable. To project raw data to a universe (our sample balancing target) we need to know the size and composition of that larger market reality…but we don't.

Sample balancing in a consumer study is manageable, because we are dealing with a person as the fundamental statistical unit. The Census Bureau produces the national demographic targets that we need to aim for, so we can "weight" individual respondents (people) by gender, age, income, geography, etc. In a retail environment, where the store is the fundamental unit of statistical analysis, certainty dissolves into chaos -- because there is no comprehensive Retail Census of all distribution channels. How much weight do we assign a single Tennis store? A Tennis Pro Shop in a country club? A Tennis department at Sports Authority? At Wal-Mart? We'll probably never know… To buyers of POS research, caveat emptor!

* * *

CHAPTER 32

A CONSUMER MAIL PANEL RESEARCH METHODOLOGY FOR SURVEYING ETHNIC POPULATIONS

Ethnic populations have always posed special challenges for survey research. A <u>minor</u> obstacle is that Blacks and Hispanics are severely underrepresented in consumer mail panels; but because panels are so large, this first problem is easily solved. Through a simple, commonplace function of "weighting" or "sample balancing", deficient groups are easily restored to their true values in the population. (If for example, we have only a third of the requisite number of Blacks in our sample, then each Black respondent is assigned a weight of three).

The second problem is more complex. When compared with their "real world" counterparts, ethnic minorities recruited for mail panels tend to be more literate, consumer-savvy, upscale and in general, more "mainstream". In a word, Black and Hispanic mail panel members do not reflect their true ethnicity, because lower income, less educated Inner City residents are not easily recruited as mail panel respondents. To compound the problem, a fundamental condition of mail panel participation is literacy in English -- a requirement that automatically excludes significant numbers of both legal and undocumented immigrants of all nationalities. Indeed, while Asians are generally more upscale than even mainstream Whites, language impediments may hinder this group's mail panel membership -- especially for older constituents. Among Hispanics, the problem is far more acute.

For all these reasons, American Sports Data, Inc. some years ago ceased tabulation and publication of ethnic sports participation statistics. In 2005 however, when resources permitted a new methodology (a diverse, cherry-picked oversample of minority populations that within certain caveats would be nationally representative) ethnic projections of sports participation in the U.S. -- at least on a one-time basis -- became feasible.

In the actual U.S. population aged six years and older, Blacks account for 11.9% of all individuals; in the TNS/NFO consumer mail panel, their presence is only 6.4%. Hispanics suffer an even greater deficiency: 14.4% in the population versus 3.8% for the panel. Asians represent only 1.5% of panel members, but 4% of the U.S. population.

Across the U.S., Black households have a median income of only $29,470, compared with $44,517 for Whites; 43% of all Black households have incomes of less than $25,000, and nearly 1 in 5 (19%) is headed by a single woman with children. Although educational attainment is on the rise, in the year 2000, only 4.8% of the Black population over age 25 held advanced degrees. For Whites, the comparable statistic for postgraduate education was 9.5%.

Descriptions vary widely, but the most convenient Census definition of Generation Y is age 5-24. Demographically, Gen Y constitutes only a small fraction of youth aged 5-24, but for the purpose of this article, they are synonymous. 34% of all Blacks are members of this age group -- an exceedingly important sports participation cohort. To the extent that young Blacks have been underrepresented in surveys, overall Black participation rates have been underestimated. This deficiency will be remedied in the present study.

Hispanics have a similar, even younger socioeconomic profile. Latino households registered a median income of only $33,565, 36% earning less than $25,000. People aged 5-24 comprise 38% of this youthful minority, which also lags Blacks in academic achievement; only 3.8% of Latinos over 35 hold advanced degrees.

But a huge unknown percentage of the U.S. Latino population speaks only Spanish. And since a precondition of consumer mail panel research is literacy (if not fluency) in English, the language gap looms as the most obvious methodological flaw in a self-administered mail survey of the Hispanic population.

The most conservative estimates place the number of undocumented Hispanics in the U.S. at 6 million: a huge "unofficial" population unrecorded in Census tabulations -- and by extension, not counted in surveys of consumer behavior. To this unknown degree, the current survey will understate projections of Hispanic sports participation.

Storied levels of educational achievement and a median household income of $55,521 raise Asian-Americans to the highest rung on the socioeconomic ladder. 17.3% hold advanced degrees, versus only 8.9% for the nation as a whole! On the other hand, a large percentage of older Asians are not fluent in English, suggesting that consumer mail panel membership (though not necessarily survey projections) may be skewed to some unknown youthful extent.

With a median household income of only $30,599 and low educational attainment, Native Americans rank near the bottom of the social hierarchy. Like other minorities, they have a substantial Gen Y contingent (37%) and a large corollary pool of sports participants; however, with only 2.5 million people (0.9% of the U.S. population) their small numbers cannot support detailed statistical segmentation in the current report.

In sum, the research challenge posed by ethnic and racial minorities is twofold: there are simply too few in consumer mail panels, and respondent profiles of successfully recruited minorities do not reflect true multicultural diversity. This first problem has a simple and straightforward solution: amass sufficient numbers of ethnic minority respondents necessary to support a minimal level of statistical analysis. With 500,000 member households, the TNS/NFO mail panel contains thousands of panelists who, when "oversampled", can easily satisfy "hard-to-fill" minority quotas that mirror the U.S. population.

Since existing Black and Hispanic mail panel members are generally far more upscale than their counterparts in the general population, the second remedy was to achieve the right "mix" of these hard-to-reach population segments: adequate proportions of Inner City residents with low income and education levels, large numbers of children, and in the case of Blacks -- a large percentage of female-headed households.

Ethnic Survey Methodology

It was decided that an augmentation of 3,000 minority questionnaires (targeted to 1,000 Blacks, 1,600 Hispanics and 400 Asians) could largely compensate for both the overall panel deficit in minorities <u>and</u> the specific shortfalls in racial mix for each group. With an oversample emphasizing youthful downscale ethnic minorities in urban settings (and also rural areas), a new expanded SUPERSTUDY® would swell to a mailout of 28,000 questionnaires.

The final step was the most crucial: to ensure that panelists who responded to the survey would be properly weighted to reflect the true composition of minority sub-groups in the U.S. population. To derive sample balancing targets, four matrices were constructed. Based on year 2000 Census data and comprised of race, age, gender, household income, market size, and region, ASD was now able to weight each respondent in the raw sample (which had been divided into 170 sub-groups) according to the degree his or her particular segment deviated from the "true" national proportion. Theoretically -- because her "type" was deficient in the sample -- a female Hispanic aged 66 might be assigned a weight of 3.25. Conversely, a Black male with an income of $35,000 from an urban area might be over-represented, and therefore receive a weight of only .85. The sample balancing variables underlying the matrices were as follows:

Defining Ourselves Through Sports Participation

Race	Gender	Age	Household Income
White	Male	6-11	<$25,000
Black	Female	12-17	$25,000-$49,999
(Non-Hispanic)		18-34	$50,000 - $74,999
Hispanic		35-54	$75,000+
Asian		55+	
Other			

Market Size	Geographic Region
<100,000	Northeast
100,000 - 1,999,999	North Central
2,000,000+	South
	West

A sufficiency of female-headed Black households (and their distribution) precluded the need for sample balancing on this variable.

Since children under 18 cannot be assigned an educational "attainment" level, a sample containing younger age groups cannot be balanced on this variable. However, household income generally serves as an excellent proxy for education, and the survey is not likely to suffer from this potential imbalance.

In sum, language barriers pose the far more serious issue in consumer surveys. Legions of undocumented, youthful Hispanic "aliens" who escape the Census may severely understate the absolute projected numbers of Hispanic sports participants.

* * *

CHAPTER 33

YOU SAY EVOLUTION, I SAY DEVOLUTION
(Quirk's Marketing Research Review -- July/August 2005)

Since its inception during the first half of the 20th century, there has been a marked evolution -- some say devolution -- in marketing research data collection. It has been argued that in each successive phase of this downward spiral, methodological purity has been sacrificed for lower cost and greater convenience.

In the beginning, there was the personal interview -- the proto-tool of modern survey research. During an innocent and pristine era of only a few decades past, legions of interviewers were dispatched on foot to conduct often lengthy, sometimes very sensitive door-to-door interviews. Americans were "taken in" by the privilege of being interviewed, and interviewers were welcomed into living rooms across the nation; the annoyance, cynicism and refusal rates would come later. In 2004, the golden age of in-person research is long gone, and while in isolated redoubts of virtue a few grizzled holdouts defend this ancient ritual, the in-home face-to-face interview is nearly extinct.

Telephone research can be traced to the 1930's, but such early usage, according to Gad Nathan of Hebrew University, was to augment other forms of research. The notorious Literary Digest survey of 1936 (which incorrectly predicted a landslide by Landon over Roosevelt) has been wrongly attributed to the telephone survey. Although the sample was selected from a list of telephone owners, the ill-fated study was actually conducted by mail.

With the ubiquity of the telephone came the phone survey -- a medium that would dramatically reduce the cost of research. In 1970, U.S. household telephone penetration reached 88% -- sufficient to appease journeymen, but not purists. But by the 1980's, the heir-apparent to personal interviewing -- righteously cloaked in the robe of Random Digit Dialing -- had effectively dealt its progenitor the coup-de-grace. Telephone research had subverted all the defenses of the face-to-face method: it was much cheaper, and remarkably -- especially in light of its present troubles and rapid decay -- the telephone was achieving <u>higher</u> cooperation rates than its predecessor! The only disadvantage of the telephone interview was survey length; a live interrogator could remain in someone's living room for an hour-and-a-half, but most telephone respondents would not tolerate impositions in excess of 30 minutes.

Timelines are murky and overlapping, but at some point in the power struggle, the heir was forced to abdicate. Researchers ingeniously shifted the burden of data collection to the respondent, who was persuaded to fill out questionnaires on the kitchen table, dutifully return them to the company, which -- having eliminated the expense of a human interviewer -- could now perform research at a fraction of even telephone cost. Thus was the consumer mail panel born, circa 1946. Exact birthdays aside, it is safe to say that consumer mail panels (very different from "cold" mail surveys) came of age after the heyday of telephone research. It may also be safe to say that in 2004 -- despite the encroachment of the Internet and a small annual erosion of response rates -- consumer mail panels are only slightly past their prime...but the cascade has begun.

The fourth generation of this pedigree is online research. Cheaper than even the mail panel (entrepreneurs have repealed interview labor, data entry, printing and postage costs!) this state-of-the-art genre is a bonanza so huge, it threatens traditional research standards and propriety. Like all other data collection methodologies, online research has its place; but because of severe structural flaws and an Internet usage rate below 70%, this futuristic technique cannot yet lay claim to nationally projectable samples. Nonetheless, we see more cavalier and more frequent references to "national surveys", where unfastidious researchers -- innocently abetted by journalists -- omit the caveat of non-projectability, inflicting a gigantic hoax on the American public. Astonishingly, the perpetrators are seldom if ever challenged. Still worse, members of online research panels -- lured and continuously motivated by prizes and economic incentives -- are highly self-selected: atypical even of the Internet users they purport to represent.

Unduly harsh critics add that this instantaneous, speed-of-light technique encourages sloppiness, methodological looseness and impropriety -- backsliding trends in survey research that parallel the rise of Generation Y, and as a more general proposition, the erosion of American cultural and business values.

In an abrupt, manic swing toward the _virtues_ of Internet research, we can also speak about the eventual dominance of the method: it is by far the most agreeable survey-taking experience, and numerous other advantages practically ensure that long before it deserves the honor, online panel research will receive the imprimatur of legitimacy. As telephone penetration achieved 88% in 1970 and became acceptable to generalists, so may the online method one day achieve universal respectability -- but not before it reaches the 90% penetration level, and certainly not before overhauling its infrastructure. But as a leading-edge tool for the conduct of "boutique" research <u>not requiring projectability</u>, (individual Health Club surveys for example) online research has already proved invaluable.

Personal Interviewing

The personal interview belongs to a recent but already mythic era of American history. Only four or five decades old, this near-perfect slice of Americana, iconized by "Father Knows Best", "Leave it to Beaver" and "Betty Crocker" -- was by nature, very friendly to an immature marketing research industry. Parents, bosses and teachers were feared, the work ethic abided and civility respected; and by today's standards, honesty remained a cherished value. The innocent culture that required suitably dressed families to regularly dine together also insisted that retail customers be fawned over; and by complex extension, naïve Americans somehow condoned the mass invasion of their living rooms by armies of hired personal interviewers.

These were the salad days of research, when communities were safe, homes accessible, respondents agreeable. People were flattered by the opportunity to serve as research subjects, and it may have even been possible to select and interview a true random population sample -- where all people in the U.S. had an equal chance of being heard. But in 2004, "probability" samples are lost to antiquity and research mythology.

In a classical face-to-face interview for example, people even then may have been a little embarrassed about sedentary behavior; chances are the method resulted in some exaggeration of active sports and fitness participation levels. And when "under-the-gun" of a live interviewer, people undoubtedly exaggerated the <u>frequency</u> of sports participation -- how many days per year they engaged in various sports and activities.

But all these questions are moot, because the personal interview is now an archaic curiosity -- fossilized by prohibitive cost, security fears, gated communities, high-rise buildings, Inner-City inaccessibility, working women, harried lifestyles, and more recently -- a heightened sensitivity to personal intrusion.

Telephone Interviewing

Telephone interviews could be conducted at a fraction of the former cost, and while they eventually became respectable, they had to be brief: a survey of more than 30 minutes ran the risk of being aborted. Another disadvantage of the telephone was that for questions demanding careful thought, contemplation (or even simple calculation!) respondents were impossibly <u>rushed</u>, and could not pause for a moment as they might during a personal interview. A mail or online questionnaire by contrast, allows unlimited meditation.

Although people are more willing to discuss sensitive matters on the phone, there is still inhibition and reticence. Even on the phone, the influence and pressure of a live interviewer is still palpable -- a limitation of both telephone and personal interviewing to which the private, anonymous mail or Internet survey is immune.

In recent years, cell phones, voicemail, multiple land lines, telemarketing "research" scams, no-call lists, working women and general time constraints have all conspired against the telephone method. With the possible exception of extravagantly-funded government research featuring unlimited callbacks, a net completion rate of 30% may be the norm. This helps explain why, after years of slower depredation by consumer mail panels, the telephone sector is being smashed to pieces by the juggernaut of online research.

All things considered, telephone surveying is not the methodology of choice for sports participation. Interviews are too brief to cover a wide range of sports, and when under the extreme pressure of a phone interview, people become unnerved and susceptible to all manner of memory distortion.

Consumer Mail Panel Research

The next watershed was the consumer mail panel. In this paradigm shift, literally millions of cooperative respondents (drawn from the ranks of ordinary households) were recruited to answer self-administered mail questionnaires on a variety of subjects generally (but not exclusively) related to consumer products and marketing. As of 2004, the three major consumer mail operators in the U.S. -- TNS-NFO, NPD and Synovate have aggregate offline panels totaling over a million American households. But this number is withering before the onslaught of Internet methodology.

While panelists are usually given incentives for longer, more tedious or unusual questionnaires, financial gain is <u>not</u> a main motive for membership -- a monumental distinction between the mail method and its online successor. Mail panelists are generally "product-oriented", enjoying free samples of new, not-yet-released offerings, or otherwise being on the leading edge of consumer marketing research. When compared with non-panel households, they are also more educated, literate, and upscale. Roughly 5% of American households can be recruited for consumer mail panels, but -- quite fortuitously -- this apparent lack of representation does not disqualify the methodology from producing valid, national projections of consumer behavior. Indeed, the well-known and highly respected Consumer Confidence Survey is based on mail panel methodology. Pre-recruited consumer mail panels generally yield 50% - 70% response rates, compared with only 5% - 20% for "cold" mail surveys of the general population...even when the latter are seeded with generous incentives.

Detractors of the method insist that a swath of panel members cannot represent a true sample of the U.S. population. On its face, this is a convincing argument; upon greater magnification, it becomes spurious. The ideal of survey research is a miniature replica of the larger reality; but academic purists, untutored research salesmen hawking competitive methodologies and other fuzzy thinkers incorrectly believe that to execute a valid survey, the <u>characteristics</u> of a sample must <u>match</u> those of the larger universe. The mail panel member, they argue, is too "queer a duck" for this purpose.

Ideally, it is desirable for a sample to clone the larger universe, but <u>this is not an absolute precondition</u> -- if the measured phenomena (in this case, sports participation behavior) are found to be <u>similar or identical in both groups</u>. Very simply, certain characteristics of a sample may be different from those in the universe it tries to mimic; but despite these differences, both populations exhibit similar behaviors. After the usual sample balancing weights are applied, the rates of sports and fitness participation behavior among panel members are similar to those in non-panel households -- a concordance first observed in the 1980's between ASD mail panel surveys and the celebrated Gallup poll. While panel and non-panel households may differ on a single issue -- the willingness to join a mail panel -- they can be (and are) highly compatible in other attitudes and behaviors. <u>Sample bias need not translate to results bias</u>; and differences in panel member composition notwithstanding, consumer mail panels are a perfectly viable methodology for sports participation research. In fact, when advantages of all methods are weighed and credited, consumer mail panel research could even emerge as the preferred methodology. But preferences of 2004 have no claim to immortality.

The Achilles Heel of mail research is a lack of control over the respondent. A physical interviewer -- either on the phone or in the flesh -- ensures that the proper household member responds to (and understands) each and every question. In a mail survey of any kind, respondents -- for reasons of disinterest, fatigue, mischief, laziness or any other reason -- may, quite whimsically, skip items in a long battery, ignore parts of a question, or simply answer a survey in a sloppy, haphazard manner. Deliberate sabotage is rare, but unless controls are in place, less-than-scrupulous respondent behavior can distort the results of a mail study.

In mail panel parlance, recent recruits ("Eager Beavers") tend to be more conscientious than are some seasoned panelists ("Lazy Dogs"). So in a tracking study, one needs from year to year, to include identical proportions of fresh, enthusiastic panel members and their more experienced counterparts -- especially the bored and disaffected. Through a form of sample balancing targeted to a base year -- in this case the use of "panel tenure" (the number of years each respondent has been a panel member) as a weighting variable -- the researcher can control for this type of response "decay".

When people respond to mail surveys in a diligent and meticulous manner (and if controls are in place to guard against those who do not), the net quantity and quality of information provided for sports and fitness participation can equal or surpass that of any other data collection method. The key advantages of self-administered questionnaires of any type, and for any subject, are:

- The ability to collect <u>more information</u>. It enables the measurement of many sports -- far more than would be possible in telephone, and even face-to-face interviews. The ASD SUPERSTUDY® of Sports Participation, monitors 103 sports/activities in a single questionnaire.

- A more relaxed, unpressured environment allows the respondent to provide <u>more thoughtful and considered answers</u>; for numerical recall, this advantage is monumental. When asked by a phone or personal interviewer how many years he or she has participated in a given sport/activity (or the number of times per year), the interviewee is on the spot -- he or she must *instantly* blurt out a number. But in the solitude and serenity of a kitchen table, family room or den, people can quietly ponder such questions, and provide much better (if still imperfect) written answers.

- A private, anonymous setting, shielded from the influence/intimidation of a human interviewer, also evokes far <u>more candid responses</u> -- especially when the material is sensitive, potentially embarrassing or threatening. In a live interview, a respondent might not confess true bodyweight or sedentary behavior; but a self-administered questionnaire could topple these inhibitions.

- The reasonable assurance that <u>panelists are not "in it for the money"</u>.

Online Research

Online research is the new frontier of data collection methodology, a fourth milestone following in-person, telephone and mail panel interviewing. Modeled after the consumer mail panel, the phenomenon of online research (or some variation thereof) may be the final paradigm, destined to supercede all traditional forms of direct consumer data collection. Like all great technological revolutions, the new methodology offers untold possibilities -- for better or worse.

With over 65% of all U.S. households having Internet access, and a much higher penetration rate among young people (who still represent the prime sporting goods market segments) online panel research is becoming an increasingly attractive tool for sports marketing studies. When "projectability" is not a requirement, its potential increases logarithmically. But the self-selected composition of an online panel will always be a lingering question-mark; and to the degree that online panelists are thought to be prize-motivated, the question becomes serious, if not insuperable.

Online panel research has inherited some, not all virtues of the offline method; but the virtual abolition of both questionnaire mailing and printing expense makes this new technique considerably less costly than its pencil-and-paper forerunner. However, online panel operators have not yet passed this theoretical savings onto their clients; in many cases, when completed interviews and data collection volume are equalized, Internet research -- ostensibly due to front-end programming costs, but also because of huge incentives -- proves <u>more expensive</u> than its older, hardcopy rival.

Like the consumer snail-mail method, online surveys may capture relatively large amounts of information while providing a quiet, anonymous setting. Unlike its glacial predecessor -- which relied on the U.S. Postal Service -- this emerging research technology can deliver huge study samples almost instantaneously.

Gargantuan online panels (5+ million members!) allow researchers access to low-incidence, hard-to-find populations such as Treadmill buyers or Big-Game Hunters of a particular species; but on the other hand, the Internet is still an exclusive club, which continues to bar certain groups. For example, the large offline population of "Bubbas" (the psychographic most fond of Hunting) is denied representation in an online study, creating an incomplete and unpromising sports participation research venue for that industry.

Returning to incomparable <u>advantages</u> of the Internet: the availability of graphics, video and audio clips -- features invaluable to concept tests, market studies and product-focused research. Add to this other forms of visual enjoyment, ease-of-operation, further control over the respondent, the dominance of online research seems almost inevitable.

Most critically, the online method silences a major objection to hardcopy mail research: it can force an answer to each and every question in a survey -- potentially <u>the greatest single advantage of Internet research over the mail method</u>. But as Don Dillman of Washington State University has suggested, this "benefit" has a double edge: it could irritate prize-happy respondents who are racing to the "submit" button, accentuating slovenly response practices.

When panelists remain true to the mission, good research is possible. But the monetary lure reigns supreme, and to the extent that respondents deviate from the straight-and-narrow, economically-based recruitment and frequently-used incentives become major structural flaws of online panel methodology. Technology and economic incentives may be transforming a pool of once-diligent, civic-minded respondents into a horde of game-playing prize-seekers who view questionnaires and survey content as a necessary evil -- an annoying obstacle to a grand prize, to be dispatched as quickly as possible. In this new paradigm, says Dillman, "the implied social contract between researcher and

You say Evolution, I say Devolution

respondent" has been fundamentally altered.

For any attitudinal, behavioral or public opinion measurement in which online and offline populations differ significantly, there can be no valid claim to national projectability -- regardless of any "algorithms" or "weights" which purport to "adjust" the data. "Balancing" an online sample by using Census demographics of the "entire" U.S. is -- quite euphemistically -- a fandangle. This is because the *offline* population (other 30%) is a vastly different breed; the attitudes and behaviors of an unwired population cannot be divined from its "wired" counterparts.

Defenders of online research disagree, however. They point to comparisons with other methods, where similarities have been found on a wide range of topics, such as the incidence of specific medical conditions, or the general consumption of mass market commodities, e.g. toothpaste or cereal. But some of these claims are specious, because Internet access is <u>not</u> a defining characteristic of such general conditions or mass market behaviors. It comes as no surprise (and proves nothing!) that razor blade purchases may not differ significantly between online and offline populations.

When Internet usage correlates strongly with lifestyle or some core element of attitude or behavior, the two populations diverge rather sharply. ASD experimental research has confirmed for example, that males 18-34 with online access have much higher sports participation rates than offline members of the same demographics, even <u>after</u> all other factors (especially income) have been held constant. At first glance, it seems counterintuitive that Internet users are _more_ active than their offline counterparts. But the online population is also younger, more affluent and better-educated than those without access to the Internet; so it is not unexpected that the former are prone to be more active in sports/fitness participation.

In any event, the flimsiest pretext of valid "projectable" online data requires ongoing, cost-prohibitive, parallel tracking research; and even then, such a claim would be highly questionable.

As Internet penetration approaches 90% - 95%, the problem will recede, and only when recruitment/incentive strategies are reconsidered will it eventually disappear…One day there will be valid, national online surveys; but that day is far off. Right now, if they must write about such things, journalists should use a much more scrupulous description of interactive research: "a nationally representative survey of a highly self-selected element of the U.S. *online* population".

* * *

APPENDIX:

THE SUPERSTUDY® OF

SPORTS PARTICIPATION

(1987-2004)

THE SUPERSTUDY® OF SPORTS PARTICIPATION

U.S. Population -- 6 Years and Older
* at least once in last 12 months*
(thousands of people)

FITNESS ACTIVITIES GENERAL	1987 Benchmark	1990	1993	1998	2000	2002	2003	2004	1-Year Change 2003-2004	6-year Change 1998-2004	17-Year Change 1987-2004
Aerobics (High-Impact)	13,961	12,359	10,356	7,460	5,581	5,423	5,875	5,521	-6.0%[t]	-26.0%	-60.5%
Aerobics (Low-Impact)	11,888	15,950	13,418	12,774	9,752	9,286	8,813	8,493	-3.6%[t]	-33.5%	-28.6%
Aerobics (Step)	n.a.	n.a.	11,502	10,784	8,963	8,336	8,457	8,257	-2.4%[t]	-23.4%	-28.2%[2]
Aerobics (Net)	21,225	23,015	24,839	21,017	17,326	16,046	16,451	15,767	-4.2%[t]	-25.0%	-25.7%
Other Exercise to Music	n.a.	n.a.	n.a.	13,846	12,337	13,540	14,159	16,365	+15.6%	+18.2%	n.a.
Aquatic Exercise	n.a.	n.a.	n.a.	6,685	6,367	6,995	7,141	5,812	-18.6%	-13.1%	n.a.
Calisthenics	n.a.	n.a.	n.a.	30,982	27,790	26,862	28,007	25,562	-8.7%	-17.5%	n.a.
Cardio Kickboxing	n.a.	n.a.	n.a.	n.a.	7,163	5,940	5,489	4,773	-13.0%	n.a.	-33.4%[6]
Fitness Bicycling	n.a.	n.a.	n.a.	13,556	11,435	11,153	12,048	10,210	-15.3%	-24.7%	n.a.
Fitness Walking	27,164	37,384	36,325	36,395	36,207	37,981	37,945	40,299	+6.2%	+10.7%	+48.4%
Gymnastics	n.a.	n.a.	n.a.	6,224	6,689	5,149	5,189	5,273	+1.6%[t]	-15.3%	n.a.
Running/Jogging	37,136	35,722	34,057	34,962	33,680	35,866	36,152	37,310	+3.2%[t]	+6.7%	+0.5%[t]
Fitness Swimming	16,912	18,045	17,485	15,258	14,060	14,542	15,899	15,636	-1.7%[t]	+2.5%[t]	-7.5%
Pilates Training	n.a.	n.a.	n.a.	n.a.	1,739	4,671	9,469	10,541	+11.3%	n.a.	+506.2%[6]
Stretching	n.a.	n.a.	n.a.	35,114	36,408	38,367	42,096	40,799	-3.1%[t]	+16.2%	n.a.
Yoga/Tai Chi	n.a.	n.a.	n.a.	5,708	7,400	11,106	13,371	12,414	-7.2%	+117.5%	n.a.

Appendix

THE SUPERSTUDY® OF SPORTS PARTICIPATION
U.S. Population -- 6 Years and Older
at least once in last 12 months
(thousands of people)

FITNESS ACTIVITIES (Continued)

EQUIPMENT EXERCISE	1987 Benchmark	1990	1993	1998	2000	2002	2003	2004	1-Year Change 2003-2004	6-year Change 1998-2004	17-Year Change 1987-2004
Barbells	n.a.	n.a.	n.a.	21,263	21,972	24,812	25,645	24,103	-6.0%	+13.4%	n.a.
Dumbbells	n.a.	n.a.	n.a.	23,414	25,241	28,933	30,549	31,415	+2.8%(†)	+34.2%	n.a.
Hand Weights	n.a.	n.a.	n.a.	23,325	27,086	28,453	29,720	30,143	+1.4%(†)	+29.2%	n.a.
Free Weights (Net)	22,553	26,728	28,564	41,266	44,499	48,261	51,567	52,056	+0.9%(†)	+26.1%	+130.8%
Weight/Resistance Machines	15,261	16,776	19,446	22,519	25,182	27,848	29,996	30,903	+3.0%(†)	+37.2%	+102.5%
Home Gym Exercise	3,905	4,748	6,258	7,577	8,103	8,924	9,260	9,347	+0.9%(†)	+23.4%	+139.4%
Abdominal Machine/Device	n.a.	n.a.	n.a.	16,534	18,119	17,370	17,364	17,440	+0.4%(†)	+5.5%(†)	n.a.
Rowing Machine Exercise	14,481	14,639	11,263	7,485	6,229	7,092	6,484	7,303	+12.6%	-2.4%(†)	-49.6%
Stationary Cycling (Upright Bike)	n.a.	n.a.	n.a.	20,744	17,894	17,403	17,488	17,889	+2.3%(†)	-13.8%	n.a.
Stationary Cycling (Spinning)	n.a.	n.a.	n.a.	6,776	5,431	6,135	6,462	6,777	+4.9%(†)	0	n.a.
Stationary Cycling (Recumbent Bike)	n.a.	n.a.	n.a.	6,773	8,947	10,217	10,683	11,227	+5.1%(†)	+65.8%	n.a.
Stationary Cycling (Net)	30,765	39,823	35,975	30,791	28,795	29,083	30,952	31,431	+1.6%(†)	+2.1%(†)	+2.8%(†)
Treadmill Exercise	4,396	11,484	19,685	37,073	40,816	43,431	45,572	47,463	+4.1%	+28.0%	+979.7%
Stair-Climbing Machine Exercise	2,121	13,498	22,494	18,609	15,828	14,251	14,321	13,300	-7.1%(†)	-28.5%	+527.1%

THE SUPERSTUDY® OF SPORTS PARTICIPATION
U.S. Population – 6 Years and Older
* at least once in last 12 months*
(thousands of people)

FITNESS ACTIVITIES (Continued)

EQUIPMENT EXERCISE (Continued)	1987 Benchmark	1990	1993	1998	2000	2002	2003	2004	1-Year Change 2003-2004	6-year Change 1998-2004	17-Year Change 1987-2004
Aerobic Rider	n.a.	n.a.	n.a.	5,868	3,817	3,654	2,955	2,468	-16.5%(†)	-57.9%	n.a.
Elliptical Motion Trainer	n.a.	n.a.	n.a.	3,863	6,176	10,695	13,415	15,678	+16.9%	+305.9%	n.a.
Cross-Country Ski Machine Exercise	n.a.	6,390	9,792	6,870	5,444	5,074	4,744	4,155	-12.4%(†)	-39.5%	-35.0%(1)

(1) 14-Year Change
(2) 11-Year Change
(3) 7-Year Change
(5) 5-Year Change
(6) 4-Year Change
(8) 2-Year Change

(†) Statistically Insignificant Change at 95% Confidence Level

Appendix

THE SUPERSTUDY® OF SPORTS PARTICIPATION

U.S. Population -- 6 Years and Older
* at least once in last 12 months*
(thousands of people)

RECREATIONAL SPORTS/ACTIVITIES

TEAM SPORTS	1987 Benchmark	1990	1993	1998	2000	2002	2003	2004	1-Year Change 2003-2004	6-year Change 1998-2004	17-Year Change 1987-2004
Baseball	15,098	15,454	15,586	12,318	10,881	10,402	10,885	9,694	-10.4%	-21.3%	-35.8%
Basketball	35,737	39,808	42,138	42,417	37,552	36,584	35,439	34,223	-3.4%[t]	-19.3%	-4.2%[t]
Cheerleading	n.a.	3,039	3,257	3,266	3,377	3,596	3,574	4,131	+15.6%[t]	+26.5%	+35.9%[t]
Ice Hockey	2,393	2,762	3,204	2,915	2,761	2,612	2,789	1,998	-28.4%	-31.5%	-16.5%
Field Hockey	n.a.	n.a.	n.a.	1,375	1,349	1,096	n.a.	n.a.	n.a.	n.a.	n.a.
Football (Touch)	20,292	20,894	21,241	17,382	15,456	14,903	14,119	12,993	-8.0%[t]	-25.3%	-36.0%
Football (Tackle)	n.a.	n.a.	n.a.	n.a.	5,673	5,783	5,751	5,440	-5.4%[t]	n.a.	-4.1%[6]
Football (Net)	n.a.	n.a.	n.a.	n.a.	18,285	18,703	17,958	16,436	-8.5%	n.a.	-10.1%[6]
Lacrosse	n.a.	n.a.	n.a.	926	751	921	1,132	914	-19.3%[t]	-1.3%[t]	n.a.
Rugby	n.a.	n.a.	n.a.	546	n.a.	n.a.	n.a.	n.a.	n.a.	n.a.	n.a.
Soccer (Indoor)	n.a.	n.a.	n.a.	n.a.	n.a.	n.a.	4,563	4,349	-4.7%[t]	n.a.	n.a.
Soccer (Outdoor)	n.a.	n.a.	n.a.	n.a.	n.a.	n.a.	16,133	14,608	-9.4%	n.a.	n.a.
Soccer (Net)	15,388	15,945	16,365	18,176	17,734	17,641	17,679	15,900	-10.1%	-12.5%	+3.3%[t]

THE SUPERSTUDY® OF SPORTS PARTICIPATION

U.S. Population – 6 Years and Older
* at least once in last 12 months*
(thousands of people)

RECREATIONAL SPORTS/ACTIVITIES
(Continued)

TEAM SPORTS (Continued)

	1987 Benchmark	1990	1993	1998	2000	2002	2003	2004	1-Year Change 2003-2004	6-year Change 1998-2004	17-Year Change 1987-2004
Softball (Regular)	n.a.	n.a.	n.a.	19,407	17,585	14,372	14,410	14,267	-1.0%[t]	-26.5%	n.a.
Softball (Fast-Pitch)	n.a.	n.a.	n.a.	3,702	3,795	3,658	3,487	4,042	+15.9%[t]	+9.2%[t]	n.a.
Softball (Net)	n.a.	n.a.	n.a.	21,352	19,668	16,587	16,020	16,324	+1.9%[t]	-23.5%	n.a.
Volleyball (Hard Surface)	n.a.	n.a.	n.a.	n.a.	n.a.	11,748	11,008	11,762	+6.8%[t]	n.a.	+0.1%[t][8]
Volleyball (Grass)	n.a.	n.a.	n.a.	n.a.	n.a.	8,621	7,953	9,163	+15.2%	n.a.	+6.3%[t][8]
Volleyball (Beach)	n.a.	11,560	13,509	10,572	8,763	7,516	7,454	7,741	+3.9%[t]	-26.8%	-33.0%[t]
Volleyball (Net)	35,984	39,633	37,757	26,637	22,876	21,488	20,286	22,216	+9.5%	-16.6%	-38.3%

RACQUET SPORTS

	1987 Benchmark	1990	1993	1998	2000	2002	2003	2004	1-Year Change 2003-2004	6-year Change 1998-2004	17-Year Change 1987-2004
Badminton	14,793	13,559	11,908	9,936	8,490	6,765	5,937	6,432	+8.3%[t]	-35.3%	-56.5%
Platform Tennis	n.a.	n.a.	n.a.	352	n.a.	n.a.	n.a.	n.a.	n.a.	n.a.	n.a.
Racquetball	10,395	9,213	7,412	5,853	5,155	4,840	4,875	5,533	+13.5%	-5.5%[t]	-46.8%
Squash	n.a.	n.a.	n.a.	289	364	302	473	290	-38.7%[t]	0	n.a.
Tennis	21,147	21,742	19,346	16,937	16,598	16,353	17,325	18,346	+5.9%[t]	+8.3%	-13.2%

Appendix

THE SUPERSTUDY® OF SPORTS PARTICIPATION

U.S. Population -- 6 Years and Older
* at least once in last 12 months*
(thousands of people)

RECREATIONAL SPORTS/ACTIVITIES (Continued)	1987 Benchmark	1990	1993	1998	2000	2002	2003	2004	1-Year Change 2003-2004	6-year Change 1998-2004	17-Year Change 1987-2004
INDIVIDUAL CONTACT SPORTS											
Boxing	n.a.	n.a.	n.a.	n.a.	1,085	908	945	1,140	+20.6%(†)	n.a.	+5.1%(†)(6)
Martial Arts	n.a.	n.a.	n.a.	5,368	5,722	5,996	6,883	6,898	+0.2%(†)	+28.5%	n.a.
Wrestling	n.a.	n.a.	n.a.	n.a.	2,405	2,026	1,820	2,303	+26.5%	n.a.	-4.2%(†)(6)
INDOOR GAMES											
Billiards/Pool	35,297	38,862	40,254	39,654	37,483	39,527	40,726	36,356	-10.7%	-8.3%	+3.0%(†)
Bowling	47,823	53,537	49,022	50,593	53,844	53,160	55,035	53,603	-2.6%(†)	+5.9%	+12.1%
Darts	n.a.	n.a.	n.a.	21,792	18,484	19,703	19,486	n.a.	n.a.	n.a.	n.a.
Table Tennis	n.a.	20,089	17,689	14,999	13,797	12,796	13,511	14,286	+5.7%(†)	-4.7%(†)	-28.9%(†)
SKATING SPORTS											
Roller Hockey	n.a.	n.a.	2,323	3,876	3,287	2,875	2,718	1,788	-34.2%	-53.9%	-23.0%(2)
Roller Skating (2x2 Wheels)	n.a.	27,101	24,223	14,752	10,834	10,968	11,746	11,103	-5.5%(†)	-24.7%	-59.0%(1)
Roller Skating (In-Line Wheels)	n.a.	4,695	13,689	32,010	29,024	21,572	19,233	17,348	-9.8%	-45.8%	+269.5%(1)
Scooter Riding (Non-Motorized)	n.a.	n.a.	n.a.	n.a.	13,881	13,858	11,493	10,196	-11.3%	n.a.	-26.5%(6)
Skateboarding	n.a.	9,267	5,388	7,190	11,649	12,997	11,090	10,592	-4.5%(†)	+47.3%	-2.7%(†)
Ice Skating	10,888	n.a.	n.a.	18,710	17,496	14,530	17,049	14,692	-13.8%	-21.5%	n.a.

- 323 -

THE SUPERSTUDY® OF SPORTS PARTICIPATION

U.S. Population – 6 Years and Older
at least once in last 12 months
(thousands of people)

RECREATIONAL SPORTS/ACTIVITIES (Continued)

STREET SPORTS

	1987 Benchmark	1990	1993	1998	2000	2002	2003	2004	1-Year Change 2003-2004	6-Year Change 1998-2004	17-Year Change 1987-2004
Stickball	n.a.	n.a.	n.a.	423	n.a.	n.a.	n.a.	n.a.	n.a.	n.a.	n.a.
Street Hockey	n.a.	n.a.	n.a.	3,601	2,448	n.a.	n.a.	n.a.	n.a.	n.a.	n.a.
Double Dutch	n.a.	n.a.	n.a.	n.a.	n.a.	n.a.	n.a.	1,558	n.a.	n.a.	n.a.

OTHER RECREATIONAL ACTIVITIES

	1987 Benchmark	1990	1993	1998	2000	2002	2003	2004	1-Year Change 2003-2004	6-Year Change 1998-2004	17-Year Change 1987-2004
Bicycling (BMX)	n.a.	n.a.	n.a.	n.a.	3,977	3,885	3,365	2,642	-21.5%	n.a.	n.a.
Bicycling (Recreational)	n.a.	n.a.	n.a.	54,575	53,006	53,524	53,710	52,021	-3.1%[t]	-4.7%	n.a.
Fencing	n.a.	n.a.	n.a.	527	n.a.	n.a.	n.a.	n.a.	n.a.	n.a.	n.a.
Golf	26,261	28,945	28,610	29,961	30,365	27,812	27,314	25,723	-5.8%	-14.1%	-33.6%[6]
Walking (Recreational)	n.a.	n.a.	n.a.	80,864	82,561	84,986	88,799	92,677	+4.4%	+14.6%	n.a.
Paintball	n.a.	n.a.	n.a.	5,923	7,121	8,679	9,835	9,640	-2.0%[t]	+62.8%	-2.0%[t]

[1] 14-Year Change
[2] 11-Year Change
[3] 7-Year Change
[5] 5-Year Change
[6] 4-Year Change
[8] 2-Year Change

[t] Statistically Insignificant Change at 95% Confidence Level

Appendix

THE SUPERSTUDY® OF SPORTS PARTICIPATION

U.S. Population – 6 Years and Older
* at least once in last 12 months*
(thousands of people)

OUTDOORS SPORTS/ACTIVITIES

OUTDOORS	1987 Benchmark	1990	1993	1998	2000	2002	2003	2004	1-Year Change 2003-2004	6-year Change 1998-2004	17-Year Change 1987-2004
Camping (Tent)	35,232	36,915	34,772	42,677	42,241	40,316	41,891	41,561	-0.8%(†)	-2.6%(†)	+18.0%
Camping (R.V.)	22,655	20,764	22,187	18,188	19,035	18,747	19,022	17,424	-8.4%	-4.2%(†)	-23.1%
Camping (Net)	50,386	50,537	49,858	50,650	51,606	49,808	51,007	49,412	-3.1%(†)	-2.4%(†)	-1.9%(†)
Canoeing	n.a.	n.a.	n.a.	13,615	13,134	10,933	11,632	11,449	-1.6%(†)	-15.9%	n.a.
Kayaking	n.a.	n.a.	n.a.	3,501	4,137	5,562	6,324	6,147	-2.8%(†)	+75.6%	n.a.
Rafting	n.a.	n.a.	n.a.	5,570	4,941	4,431	4,553	4,209	-7.6%(†)	-24.4%	n.a.
Hiking (Day)	n.a.	n.a.	n.a.	38,629	39,015	36,778	39,096	39,334	+0.6%(†)	+1.8%(†)	n.a.
Hiking (Overnight)	n.a.	n.a.	n.a.	6,821	6,750	5,839	6,213	6,396	+2.9%(†)	-6.2%(†)	n.a.
Hiking (Net)	n.a.	n.a.	n.a.	40,117	40,133	37,888	40,409	40,713	+0.8%(†)	+1.5%(†)	n.a.
Horseback Riding	n.a.	n.a.	n.a.	16,522	16,988	14,641	16,009	14,695	-8.2%	-11.1%	n.a.
Mountain Biking	1,512	4,146	7,408	8,611	7,854	6,719	6,940	5,334	-23.1%	-38.1%	+252.8%
Mountain/Rock Climbing	n.a.	n.a.	n.a.	2,004	1,947	2,089	2,169	2,161	-0.4%(†)	+7.8%(†)	n.a.
Artificial Wall Climbing	n.a.	n.a.	n.a.	4,696	6,117	7,185	8,634	7,659	-11.3%	+63.1%	n.a.
Trail Running	n.a.	n.a.	n.a.	5,249	5,232	5,625	6,109	6,486	+6.2%(†)	+23.6%	n.a.

THE SUPERSTUDY® OF SPORTS PARTICIPATION

U.S. Population -- 6 Years and Older
at least once in last 12 months
(thousands of people)

OUTDOORS SPORTS/ACTIVITIES (Continued)

SHOOTING SPORTS	1987 Benchmark	1990	1993	1998	2000	2002	2003	2004	1-Year Change 2003-2004	6-year Change 1998-2004	17-Year Change 1987-2004
Archery	8,558	9,252	8,648	7,109	6,047	6,650	7,111	6,756	-5.0%(†)	-5.0%(†)	-21.1%
Hunting (Shotgun/Rifle)	25,241	23,220	23,189	16,684	16,481	16,471	15,232	15,196	-0.2%(†)	-8.9%	-39.8%
Hunting (Bow)	n.a.	n.a.	n.a.	4,719	4,120	4,752	4,155	3,661	-11.9%(†)	-22.4%	n.a.
Shooting (Sporting Clays)	n.a.	2,932	3,100	2,734	2,843	3,017	3,867	3,222	-16.7%	+17.8%	+9.9%(†)
Shooting (Trap/Skeet)	5,073	n.a.	n.a.	3,800	3,827	3,696	4,496	4,059	-9.7%(†)	+6.8%(†)	-20.0%
Target Shooting (Rifle)	n.a.	n.a.	n.a.	14,042	12,984	14,336	15,176	14,057	-7.4%(†)	+0.1%(†)	n.a.
Target Shooting (Handgun)*	n.a.	n.a.	n.a.	12,110	10,433	11,064	13,836*	11,932	-13.8%	-1.5%(†)	n.a.
Target Shooting (Net)*	18,947	21,840	23,498	18,330	16,293	17,558	19,788*	18,037	-8.8%	-1.6%(†)	-4.8%(†)

FISHING

Fishing (Fly)	11,359	8,039	6,598	7,269	6,581	6,034	6,033	4,623	-23.4%	-36.4%	-59.3%
Fishing (Freshwater -- Other)	50,500	53,207	50,198	45,807	44,050	42,605	43,819	39,433	-10.0%	-13.9%	-21.9%
Fishing (Saltwater)	19,646	19,087	18,490	15,671	14,710	14,874	15,221	13,453	-11.6%	-14.2%	-31.5%
Fishing (Net)	58,402	58,816	55,442	55,488	53,846	51,426	52,970	47,906	-9.6%	-13.7%	-18.0%

* 2003 measurement elevated due to change in category definition from "Pistol" to "Handgun"

Appendix

THE SUPERSTUDY® OF SPORTS PARTICIPATION

U.S. Population – 6 Years and Older
* at least once in last 12 months*
(thousands of people)

OUTDOORS SPORTS/ACTIVITIES (Continued) SNOW SPORTS	1987 Benchmark	1990	1993	1998	2000	2002	2003	2004	1-Year Change 2003-2004	6-year Change 1998-2004	17-Year Change 1987-2004
Skiing (Cross-Country)	8,344	7,292	6,489	4,728	4,613	4,080	4,171	4,007	-3.9%(†)	-15.2%	-52.0%
Skiing (Downhill)	17,676	18,209	17,567	14,836	14,749	14,249	13,633	11,971	-12.2%	-19.3%	-32.3%
Snowboarding	n.a.	2,116	2,567	5,461	7,151	7,691	7,818	7,110	-9.1%(†)	+30.2%	+236.0%(†)
Snowmobiling	n.a.	n.a.	n.a.	6,492	7,032	4,515	5,509	4,688	-14.9%	-27.8%	n.a.
Snowshoeing	n.a.	n.a.	n.a.	1,721	1,970	2,006	2,479	2,302	-7.1%(†)	+33.8%	n.a.
WATER SPORTS											
Boardsailing/Windsurfing	1,145	1,025	835	1,075	655	496	779	418	-46.3%(†)	-61.1%	-63.5%
Jet Skiing	n.a.	n.a.	n.a.	11,203	10,835	9,806	10,648	7,972	-25.1%	-28.8%	n.a.
Sailing	6,368	5,981	3,918	5,902	5,271	5,161	5,232	4,307	-17.7%	-27.0%	-32.4%
Scuba Diving	2,433	2,615	2,306	3,448	2,901	3,328	3,215	3,430	+6.7%(†)	-0.5%(†)	+41.0%
Snorkeling	n.a.	n.a.	n.a.	10,575	10,526	9,865	10,179	11,112	+9.2%(†)	+5.1%(†)	n.a.
Surfing	1,459	1,224	n.a.	1,395	2,180	1,879	2,087	1,936	-7.2%(†)	+38.8%	+32.7%

THE SUPERSTUDY® OF SPORTS PARTICIPATION

U.S. Population -- 6 Years and Older
at least once in last 12 months
(thousands of people)

OUTDOORS SPORTS/ACTIVITIES (Continued)

WATER SPORTS (Continued)	1987 Benchmark	1990	1993	1998	2000	2002	2003	2004	1-Year Change 2003-2004	6-year Change 1998-2004	17-Year Change 1987-2004
Swimming (Recreational)	n.a.	n.a.	n.a.	94,371	93,976	92,667	96,429	95,268	-1.2%(†)	+1.0%(†)	n.a.
Wakeboarding	n.a.	n.a.	n.a.	2,253	3,581	3,142	3,356	2,843	-15.3%(†)	+26.2%	n.a.
Water Skiing	19,902	19,314	16,626	10,161	10,335	8,204	8,425	6,835	-18.9%	-32.7%	-65.7%

(1) 14-Year Change
(2) 11-Year Change
(3) 7-Year Change
(5) 5-Year Change
(6) 4-Year Change
(8) 2-Year Change

(†) Statistically Insignificant Change at 95% Confidence Level

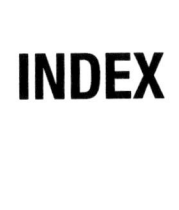

INDEX

INDEX

Abdominal Machine/Device 319
action sports 211, 237
Aerobic Rider 128, 153, 320
Aerobics (High-Impact) 187, 318
Aerobics (Low-Impact) 187, 318
Aerobics (Step) 318
after-school programs 204
anti-smoking campaign 109, 112, 175
Aquatic Exercise 61, 64, 101, 183, 318
Archery 187, 326
arthritis 84, 91
Artificial Wall Climbing 180, 186, 211, 216, 227, 230, 231, 234, 325
Asians 297, 298, 299, 301
asthma 84, 91, 130
athlete exposures 241, 244, 246, 248
athletic facilities 194, 197
attitudes and behavior 67
AYSO 197, 204, 272, 290
Baby Boomers 147, 215, 221, 237
Badminton 217, 322
Barbells 53, 64, 100, 153, 319
Baseball 20, 29, 52, 56, 181, 187, 192, 194, 202, 204, 205, 207, 212, 214, 217, 224, 236, 240, 248, 250, 261, 272, 276, 277, 321
Basketball 20, 29, 52, 56, 130, 181, 192, 197, 199, 200, 202, 203, 208, 209, 212, 217, 235, 246, 248, 250, 252, 280, 283, 284, 321

Behavioral Risk Factor Surveillance System 108, 115
best practices 205, 206
Bicycling (BMX) 62, 324
Bicycling (Recreational) 324
Billiards/Pool 217, 277, 323
Blacks 297, 298, 299, 300, 301
Blair, Stephen 135
blood sports 10, 255, 257
BMI 108, 129, 130, 134
Boardsailing 327
body mass index 43, 108, 129, 134, 135
bodyweight 16, 77, 108, 109, 111, 117, 129, 130, 132, 134, 139, 140, 161, 165, 312
Bowling 217, 262, 277, 283, 284, 323
Boxing 246, 255, 257, 323
Calisthenics 318
caloric expenditure 45, 112, 116, 126
Camping (R.V.) 186, 217, 234, 325
Camping (Tent) 217, 234, 325
Canoeing 218, 234, 285, 325
cardio equipment 148, 248
cardio exercise 59
Cardio Kickboxing 62, 65, 97, 98, 101, 184, 318
CDC 16, 43, 52, 108, 112, 115, 116, 130, 191
celebrity athletes 1, 6, 252
Census Bureau 289, 296
Centers for Disease Control 52, 108, 190
character building 155, 189
Cheerleading 194, 247, 250, 321
child obesity 133, 189

Index

cholesterol 78, 84, 91, 170, 171, 173, 175
chronic back pain 84, 88, 91
Club Business International 30, 40, 163
Comprehensive Study of Consumer Attitudes Toward Physical Fitness 79-85, 91-93, 137
Comprehensive Study of Sports Injuries in the U.S. 242, 249
confidence level 100, 128, 152, 153, 186, 187, 234, 268, 270
Consciousness I, II, III, IV 34-36, 38-40, 68-85, 105, 106, 125
Conservation and Reinvestment Act 195
consumer mail panel 55, 63, 98, 127, 131, 143, 151, 185, 215, 233, 249, 270, 285, 286, 297-299, 304, 308, 310, 312
Consumer Products Safety Commission 237, 238, 240, 242, 249
contrarian philosophies 133
counterculture 3, 5, 13, 103, 156-158, 167, 193, 215, 254
crime rate 4, 7, 109, 110, 223
Cross-Country Ski Machine Exercise 320
cultural revolution 5
Curves for Women 73, 77, 78, 125, 149, 160
Darts 323
deconditioned 59
demographics 11, 45, 60, 110, 124, 147, 221, 265, 276, 293, 315
Dewey, John 207, 209
diabetes 44, 47, 78, 84, 91, 130, 150, 170, 175
diet pills 36, 142, 144, 175
dieting 10, 36, 85, 117, 126, 139, 141, 146, 175
Double Dutch 324
Dumbbells 64, 100, 125, 149, 153, 319
eating habits 16, 37, 105, 112, 140, 144, 165, 175

Elliptical Motion Trainer 96, 128, 148, 153, 320
emergency room 191, 235, 240, 241, 244, 245, 249
ethnicity 197, 297, 300, 301
exercise equipment 42, 75, 105, 124, 168, 171, 262, 264, 265, 294, 319-320
Express Workout 149
Extreme Sports 8, 20, 21, 45, 179, 193, 194, 200, 212-215, 237, 245, 247, 252
fat and fit 33, 134-136
female fitness 12, 54, 61
female participation 194, 195
Fencing 324
Field Hockey, 321
Fishing 11, 182, 261, 264, 290, 326
Fishing (Fly) 264, 326
Fishing (Freshwater -- Other) 326
Fishing (Saltwater) 326
fitness activity 51, 60, 62, 68, 75, 104, 116, 117, 122, 123, 149, 152, 161, 184, 190, 272, 318
fitness behavior 15, 54, 68, 76, 113, 115-117, 121, 161, 232
Fitness Bicycling 62, 318
fitness boom 19, 47, 54, 107, 112, 115, 158, 159
fitness consciousness 34, 63, 67, 76, 80-85, 158, 165
fitness enthusiasts 51, 69, 97, 98, 160, 183, 232
fitness equipment 28, 96, 105, 183
fitness growth 59
fitness industry 27, 28, 32, 55, 67, 68, 98
fitness lifestyle 46, 71, 125, 232, 251
fitness movement 13, 27, 31, 46, 63, 67, 73, 74, 103, 105, 117, 122, 147, 156, 159, 161, 183, 184, 237

Index

fitness participants 35, 46, 51, 63, 72, 80, 105, 115, 121, 147, 148, 150, 153, 157, 160, 185, 275
fitness participation 1, 7, 17, 44, 67, 74, 104, 114, 115, 152, 235, 238, 265, 284, 307, 310, 311, 316
fitness phenomenon 15, 67, 147
fitness psychographic 76
fitness revolution 7, 8, 10, 13, 14, 74, 103, 115, 150, 156-158, 160, 251
Fitness Swimming 62, 318
fitness trends 42, 95, 128, 153
Fitness Walking 53, 57, 61, 62, 65, 101, 103, 123, 128, 149, 151, 153, 159, 183, 250, 318
flexibility 59, 83, 104, 140, 141
focus-on-self 156
Football (Tackle) 186, 250, 321
Football (Touch) 56, 217, 250, 321
formal diet 117, 140, 141, 144
Free Weights (Net) 128, 319
frequency of participation 281
frequent fitness participation 76, 115, 122, 152
frequent participants 15, 21, 79-81, 123, 160, 212, 235, 244, 272
future of fitness 47, 69, 96, 103-106
gender-equity 195
Generation X 214, 221-223, 256
Generation Y 2, 21, 22, 180, 221-225, 298, 305
Golf 183, 186, 194, 206, 218, 250, 261, 263, 264, 269, 271, 281, 283, 284, 294, 295, 324
Great Outdoors 9, 227-234
Gymnastics 122, 155, 186, 196, 252, 318

Hand Weights 12, 42, 53, 55, 59, 61, 64, 100, 125, 149, 151, 153, 184, 319
health and fitness 9, 12, 15, 63, 67, 68, 156, 158, 165, 191, 251
health club exercise 139-141, 144, 175
health club members 30, 31, 51, 63, 68, 75, 79-81, 103, 122, 125, 140, 145, 146, 147, 160, 183, 184, 290
health club patrons 37, 63, 77, 79-81
health club strategy 75
health food craze 13, 158
health insurance providers 167, 172
health insurance rebates 24, 44, 171-174
healthcare 15, 23, 24, 71, 104, 106, 115, 148, 164-167, 169, 171, 174, 175, 189, 201, 202
healthy lifestyle 44, 160, 167, 168, 169, 171, 172
healthy lifestyle incentives 160, 168, 172
heart disease 44, 47, 84, 91, 150
heart rate monitors 42
high-impact 53, 97, 159, 187
Hiking (Day) 234, 325
Hiking (Overnight) 234, 325
Hispanics 11, 297-299, 301
HMO's 24, 44, 121, 166, 169, 171-174
home exercise 37, 42, 75-77, 142, 144, 146, 168, 169, 175, 265
Home Gym Exercise 64, 100, 128, 153, 319
Horseback Riding 250, 325
human nature 233
humanistic evolution 3-7, 10, 12, 14, 16-19, 21, 24, 47, 67, 181, 251, 253, 255, 257, 258
Hunting 182, 187, 218, 248, 250, 251-258, 262, 283, 290, 291, 313

Index

Hunting (Bow) 182, 187, 326
Hunting (Shotgun/Rifle) 182, 326
hypertension 91, 150
Ice Hockey 205, 246, 250, 321
Ice Skating 218, 323
IHRSA 28, 41, 130, 132, 140, 144-146, 167, 168, 172
inactive 75, 165
incentives 36, 42, 43, 55, 77, 121, 140, 160, 161, 166-168, 172, 189, 305, 309, 313, 314
incentivized physical fitness 15, 68, 104
Indifferent 34, 69, 70, 72, 106
industrial revolution 22, 112, 155
injury rates 236, 237, 243, 245, 246, 249
injury research 238, 241, 242
injury surveillance systems 239
Inner City 45, 297, 300
insomnia 84, 88, 91
Insurance 44, 139, 165-174, 239, 241, 242
Jet Skiing 327
Kayaking 217, 227, 230, 234, 325
kinder, gentler exercise 12, 47, 55, 95, 97, 104, 121, 123, 124, 125, 148, 151, 160, 163, 183, 251, 252, 255
Lacrosse 192, 194, 205, 206, 212, 236, 277, 321
Latinos 198, 299
levels of fitness consciousness 67-74
Levitt, Steven 110-111, 119
Little League 21, 197, 204, 214, 252, 272
low-impact 55, 103, 159, 183, 187
magic pill 23, 33, 68, 104

mail panel research 270, 285, 286, 297, 299, 308, 310
marathon 19, 20, 158, 208, 232, 279
market research 1, 267
Martial Arts 236, 246, 250, 323
measurement error 290
Medicare 9, 17, 24, 169, 170, 174, 175
megatrend 13, 103, 151, 158, 160, 184, 251, 252
Me-Generation 8, 9, 13, 14, 157, 158
methodology 3, 116, 141, 172, 282, 283, 286, 297, 298, 308-310, 312, 314
mind-body exercise 96, 104, 122
motivation 13, 27, 32, 42, 63, 71, 75, 98, 141, 167, 172, 185
Mountain Biking 19, 180, 216, 234, 235, 237, 246, 250, 325
Mountain/Rock Climbing 216, 233, 234, 288, 325
multivariate statistical analysis 69
National Alliance for Youth Sports 191
National Electronic Injury Surveillance System 240, 241
National Federation of State High School Associations 195
National Health Interview Survey 239
National Hospital Ambulatory Medical Care Survey 240
National Human Activity Pattern Survey 282
NCAA Injury Surveillance System 240
Nestle, Marion 118
NHANES 108, 130
no-impact 55, 60, 183
Non-Believers 69, 70, 71, 72, 106
not-for-profit 197
obesity 2, 7-10, 14-17, 21, 22, 24, 33, 44, 45, 51, 105, 107-118, 121, 129-137, 139, 140, 142-146, 160, 161, 168-170, 189, 190, 202, 236, 251

Index

obesity crisis, epidemic 9, 14, 15, 16, 51, 107, 109, 110, 113, 130, 133, 134, 142, 160

obesity subculture 7, 9, 17

Obesity-Weight Control Report 140, 144-146

older Americans 116, 147-153, 237

online panel research 306, 312, 313

organized play 194, 200

outdoors consciousness 7, 9, 19, 229

outdoors exercise 37, 76, 125, 140, 144, 146, 175, 183

Outdoors Revolution 9, 227-234

overweight 9, 19, 28, 34, 52, 71, 72, 73, 74, 78, 82, 85, 105, 108, 109, 111, 113, 125, 129, 130, 133-137, 159, 165, 190, 202, 232

Paintball 11, 180, 186, 192, 194, 200, 211, 213, 216, 247, 258, 262, 282, 324

panel tenure 270, 289, 311

PE4LIFE 190

pedometer 23, 42, 168

personal interviewing 304, 308

personal trainer 15, 16, 32, 42, 68, 98, 105, 117, 122, 141, 149, 153, 161, 168, 179, 184

physical activity 15, 22, 33, 39, 43, 44, 47, 54, 67, 68, 75, 104, 109, 112, 114-117, 135, 142, 168, 190, 191, 201, 202, 206, 236

physical appearance 73, 78, 89, 93

physical education 22, 44, 51, 52, 115, 155, 189, 190, 194, 201, 202, 209, 236

physical health 59, 67, 93, 133

physical inactivity 16, 47, 113, 114, 165

Pilates 12, 38, 46, 55, 59, 60, 64, 95, 96, 98, 100, 122, 123, 128, 148, 151, 153, 160, 171, 290, 318
Platform Tennis 322
Pleasure Principle 15, 27, 32, 68, 185, 233
pop sociology 215
POS research 275, 293-296
prescription diet drugs 144
preventive healthcare 15, 24, 71, 115, 164-167, 169, 171, 174, 175
psychographic segmentation 35
psychographics 34, 221, 293
psychological stress 2, 87-93
psychology of entitlement 45, 166, 167
Public Agenda Foundation 2, 28
public health 1, 14, 29, 52, 87, 109, 112, 115, 119, 130, 133, 134, 161, 164, 175, 267
questionnaire length 289
Racquetball 159, 187, 217, 322
Rafting 218, 234, 325
recreational sports 116, 321-324
remedial healthcare 24, 164
research methodology 172, 297
respondent cooperation 287, 294
respondent recognition 284
response distortion 288
risk assessment 239, 241
Roller Hockey 323
Roller Skating (2x2 Wheels) 187, 218, 323
Roller Skating (In-Line Wheels) 216, 250, 323
Rowing Machine Exercise 128, 153, 159, 319

Index

Rugby 321
Rugged Chic 18, 228
Running/Jogging 56, 57, 62, 65, 101, 128, 153, 250, 318
Sailing 205, 327
sample balancing 287, 295, 296, 297, 301, 302, 310, 311
sampling error 268, 289
Scooter Riding (Non-Motorized) 180, 323
Scuba Diving 204, 208, 278, 327
Sector Analysis Report 196, 219
sedentary 8, 9, 19, 22, 51, 52, 71, 72, 77, 79, 81, 82, 112, 116, 155, 159, 236, 307, 312
segmentation 34, 35, 39, 68, 69, 76, 222, 300
self-discipline 9, 68, 75, 167
self-fulfillment 5, 13, 19, 71, 156, 157, 158
self-improvement 103, 157, 158,
self-motivation 15, 16, 42, 68, 160, 185
senior fitness 7, 46, 148, 160
senior participation 12, 151, 265
Shooting (Sporting Clays) 182, 187, 326
Shooting (Trap/Skeet) 182, 187, 326
Shooting Sports 2, 11, 182, 187, 251-258, 262, 326
Skateboarding 29, 52, 56, 179, 186, 192, 193, 211, 216, 225, 235, 237, 246, 250, 252, 323
Skiing (Cross-Country) 181, 186, 218, 327
Skiing (Downhill) 181, 186, 218, 246, 250, 327
smoking 7, 10, 14, 72, 74, 82, 88, 91, 109, 112, 133, 142, 164, 168, 169, 170, 175
Snorkeling 327
Snow Sports 183, 327

Snowboarding 56, 179, 181, 186, 192, 193, 200, 211, 213, 216,
          237, 246, 248, 250, 252, 261, 269, 282, 327
Snowmobiling 186, 327
Snowshoeing 180, 181, 186, 216, 327
Soccer 21, 181, 192, 194, 202, 205, 206, 236, 246, 252,
          272, 290, 321
social analysis 2, 3, 111, 214, 251
social change 165, 251, 253
social class 45, 114
social issues 254
social morality 4, 6
social theory 251, 252
social tolerance 4, 6, 8
socioeconomic 44, 111, 113, 299
sociology 3, 215
Softball 181, 186, 192, 217, 235, 236, 246, 248, 322
Softball (Fast-Pitch) 181, 186, 217, 236, 322
Softball (Regular) 322
sporting goods 1, 28, 29, 41, 52, 56, 63, 99, 127, 151, 185, 190,
          193, 215, 224, 238, 241, 242, 261, 263, 267,
          271, 272, 273, 276, 285, 293, 294, 295, 312
Sporting Goods Manufacturers Association 28, 41, 56, 63,
          99, 127, 151, 185, 190, 215
sporting goods markets 261, 263
sports celebrities 203
sports iconography 8, 18
sports injuries 8, 191, 235-250
sports injury epidemiology 1, 238, 267
sports marketing 2, 267, 273, 312
sports medicine 237, 239, 242

Index

sports research 3, 197, 265, 284
Squash 322
Stair-Climbing Machine Exercise 128, 153, 248, 319
Stationary Cycling 53, 57, 65, 148, 159, 160, 248, 319
Stationary Cycling (Recumbent Bike) 100, 148, 160, 319
Stationary Cycling (Spinning) 101, 187, 319
Stationary Cycling (Upright Bike) 101, 128, 153, 319
Stickball 324
Street Hockey 324
strength training 59, 60, 124, 155, 250
stress reduction 78, 175
Stretching 53, 59, 60, 64, 95, 100, 104, 123, 318
subsidization of preventive healthcare 167
subsidized fitness 167
Superstudy® of Sports Participation 43, 51, 55, 59, 63, 95, 98, 122, 127, 131, 140, 143, 147, 149, 151, 179, 183, 185, 193, 211, 215-218, 228, 233, 243, 249, 288, 311, 317-328
Surfing 179, 180, 186, 216, 246, 327
Surgeon General 14, 107, 108, 109, 114, 135, 142, 164
survey research 229, 232, 267, 275, 282, 290, 297, 303, 305, 309
Swimming 196, 255, 288
Swimming (Laps/Fitness) 65, 101
Swimming (Recreational) 218, 328
Table Tennis 217, 323
Target Shooting 11, 182, 218, 253, 257, 326
Target Shooting (Handgun) 326
Target Shooting (Rifle) 326

team sports 20, 21, 181. 192, 193, 194, 196, 201, 211, 212, 213, 214, 236, 321-322
technology 8, 22, 23, 43, 68, 104, 106, 112, 163, 170, 224, 313, 314
telephone research 303, 304
telescoping 277, 278, 279, 281-285, 288, 289, 293
television 22, 53, 113, 114
Tennis 56, 159, 206, 214, 217, 235, 250, 263, 272, 283, 284, 291, 296, 322
Title IX 7, 10, 195-197, 252
TNS-NFO 55, 63, 98, 127, 131, 143, 151, 185, 215, 233, 249, 298, 300, 308
tracking study 51, 56, 59, 63, 99, 127, 131, 140, 143, 151, 179, 185, 215, 233, 249, 311
traditional sports 20, 21, 192, 211-219
Trail Running 187, 217, 234, 271, 285, 325
Treadmill Exercise 53, 55, 57, 64, 97, 98, 100, 103, 123, 124, 128, 148, 153, 159, 160, 184, 186, 235, 319
USYSA 272, 290
Uninitiated Believers 34, 35, 68, 69, 72, 73, 76, 77, 78, 81, 105
vigorous activity 54, 61
Volleyball 29, 52, 56, 181, 187, 192, 217, 247, 250, 276, 288, 321
Wakeboarding 179, 186, 192, 193, 211, 216, 237, 252, 328
Walking (Recreational) 182, 217, 250, 324
war on obesity 14, 118, 129-131, 133, 135, 139, 142
war on smoking 7, 14, 133, 142
Water Skiing 218, 328

Index

weight control 29, 37, 38, 42, 52, 78, 117, 131, 132, 140, 143, 144-146, 169, 170
weight loss 37, 77, 104, 109, 139-146, 170, 171
weight management 36, 37, 141
Weight/Resistance Machines 56, 57, 64, 100, 124, 128, 153, 184, 186, 319
Windsurfing 327
Wrestling 196, 214, 248, 252, 288, 323
Yankelovich, Daniel 2, 4, 28, 156, 167
YMCA 122, 149, 155, 160
Yoga/Tai Chi 12, 38, 42, 46, 55, 59, 60, 64, 88, 95, 96, 98, 100, 123, 128, 148, 151, 153, 160, 168, 171, 183, 184, 186, 277, 318
youth culture 22, 182, 193, 211, 215, 225, 253
youth development 2, 8, 191, 193, 199-210, 213
youth sports 189-198, 199, 202, 204, 205, 236